1997 + 1991 12 approved drugs taken off the market serious effects + deaths

had

5 million dollars in sales

Health Myths

Exposed

Learn How to Avoid Deadly Health Myths-Add 10 Years to Your Life

175 weight gain

150 deaths from drug

by

Shane Ellison M.Sc.

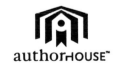

author HOUSE™

1663 LIBERTY DRIVE, SUITE 200
BLOOMINGTON, INDIANA 47403
(800) 839-8640
WWW.AUTHORHOUSE.COM

First published by AuthorHouse 11/05/04

ISBN: 1-4208-0027-2 (sc)

Library of Congress Control Number: 2004097437

Printed in the United States of America
Bloomington, Indiana

This book is printed on acid-free paper.

If a man values anything more than his health, he will eventually lose his health. The irony is that if it is comfort or wealth that he values more, he will eventually lose these too.

Table of Contents

Dedication

This book is dedicated to the FDA. Without their bias for wealth not health, this book would not have been made possible. Of course, this bias would not exist if it were not for the encouragement and financial help of the pharmaceutical industry, who pockets billions of dollars every year from the suffering of others.

Thanks

All of my thanks go to my wife and daughter for their support and encouragement in completing this book. Without it, Health Myths Exposed would not exist. In return, I hope to have taught you the importance of asking "why" in everything you do, of living for purpose and of having the courage to answer to no one but yourselves.

Also, I am thankful to the many researchers who I have learned from including, but not limited to: Edward Griffin, Uffe Ravnskov MD, PhD, Joseph Mercola DO John Hammell, Jon Rappaport, Edgar Civitello PhD and Neil Z. Miller.

Preface

Fact: Americans are taking more Food and Drug Administration (FDA) approved drugs (prescription drugs) than ever before.

Whether it's an attempt to save their patient's failing health, to give patients "what they want," or simply to help them "feel better," it is estimated that American medical doctors write an average of 10 prescriptions per person every year.[1] According to the Kaiser Family Foundation, US spending on prescription drugs has tripled between 1990 and 2001 to over $140.6 billion. If these trends continue, consumer spending on prescription drugs will top $445.9 billion dollars by the year 2012![2] That's a whopping $1,521.18 per year for every man, woman and child in the country!

Yet, despite this prescription drug "feeding frenzy," the United States ranks 12th out of the top 13 countries in regard to the health of its citizens.[3] Recognizing the fact that

---

[1]   The Henry J. Kaiser Family Foundation; "Prescription Drug Trends: A Chartbook;" July 2000.

[2]   Cohen, Jay, M.D. *Prescription Drug Use in America: The Startling Numbers And Their Implications.* http://www.medalternatives.com/articles/prescript_drug_use.html.

[3]   *Journal of the American Chemical Society,* July 26, 2000-Vol 284, No.4.

the more we spend on drugs the sicker we get, *Health Myths Exposed* was researched and written to discover the truth about FDA approved drugs and their impact on our health. This quest to uncover the truth began with one straightforward question that everyone should ask, yet few actually do, before using a prescription drug: "Are FDA approved drugs safe and effective?" As a medicinal chemist trained in drug design, I have learned how to interpret scientific data and have studied a plethora of medical journals, clinical studies and university research papers in an attempt to answer this question for you, the consumer.

My findings have led me to an undeniable conclusion: The notion that FDA approved drugs are safe and effective is an absolute health myth. Worse yet, I found that many prescription drugs were approved and released to the public by the FDA despite the fact that they were shown to be unsafe in test trials on otherwise healthy individuals! (For example: Lipitor, Prozac, Phen-Fen etc.)

The FDA's practice of approving unsafe drugs has lead millions to a lifetime of drug use. Let me explain. Users of FDA approved drugs are often forced to use other prescription drugs to offset the unpleasant and dangerous side effects associated with the initial drug. In many cases, this has meant a lifetime of drug use, which severely limits a person's functional capabilities and decreases their lifespan. Looking in the other direction, this trend is often ignored by medical doctors and is simply dismissed as "worsening health." It is as if the so-called "cure" of prescription drugs is worse than the illness itself.

While revealing this truth, I met much opposition from the professionals who were exposed to my findings. The most common argument I encountered in favor of using FDA approved drugs was that, when looking at the "big picture," the benefits derived from or the effectiveness of FDA approved drugs justified the risk. This was an ill thought-out hypothesis because I found that outside of "emergency medicine," rarely, if at all, is this true.

The majority of commonly used FDA approved drugs are absolutely ineffective in that they offer no benefit whatsoever.[4] Despite the multi-billion dollar ad campaigns, the media coverage, and the deceptively written articles found in the medical journals which praise the benefits of prescription drugs, the vast majority of drugs only work for 30-50% of the population, as confessed by Glaxo Chief Allen Roses.

While FDA approved drugs are ineffective for the majority of the population, they frequently cause numerous negative side effects and even death among their users. In fact, the health consequences of using these ineffective drugs were far more devastating than for elicit drugs, which the United States Government spends nearly $12 billion every year to "fight a war" against. [5] Yet, America's FDA approved drug problem continues to be ignored.

It could easily be concluded from my research that the entire medical and health industry was founded on deception and is motivated by an unquenchable thirst for profit. While the health industry tries to obscure this fact from the public, it is very well known among powerful health organizations such as the FDA, the American Medical Association (AMA), the National Institutes of Health (NIH) and the Centers for Disease Control (CDC). More often than not, the facts are ignored due to the financial interests of the top scientists and

---

[4]   Connor, Steve. *Glaxo chief: Our drugs do not work on most patients.* Independent.co.uk. 12/8/03.

[5]   Source: Office of National Drug Control Policy. The United States government spent over 19 billion dollars to fight a war on "illicit drugs", which were responsible for approximately 19,000 deaths, yet they have done nothing to curb the death toll from FDA approved drugs.

researchers within these organizations. When combined, this deception and thirst for profit has led to numerous health myths that are perpetuated on a daily basis in the newspaper, radio, and television ads that you see every day, in an attempt to sell FDA approved drugs to you and other unsuspecting consumers.

To expose these deadly myths, *Health Myths Exposed* was written. This book is for those who are dedicated to living healthy for life, without the use of pharmaceutical drugs. To this end, *Health Myths Exposed* offers the facts surrounding the sordid pharmaceutical industry in an easy to understand format.

Once you're armed with these facts, you will have the ability to avoid the myriad of health myths, which only exist to transform healthy people into lifetime assets of the pharmaceutical industry. It is not a stretch to say that reading *Health Myths Exposed* could be a matter of life and death...for you or someone close to you!

Health Myths Exposed marks the beginning of a much-needed war on FDA approved drugs. Get ready to be shocked, get ready to become angry; but most importantly: Get ready to learn some amazing things about yourself and how to live a healthy life...despite pharmaceutical drugs and medical doctors!

Myth #1 – FDA approved Drugs are Safe and Effective

Fact: Profit, rather than consumer safety, is the #1 priority of the modern FDA.

Before 1906, there were no laws to protect consumers from unsafe or unsanitary food packaging and processing methods. Death and illness from food poisoning was commonplace, and resulted mainly from tainted meat products and canned goods. To address and meet these sanitation needs, The Pure Food and Drug Act was passed in 1906.

This new law heralded the birth of a brand new watchdog agency: the Food and Drug Administration (FDA). During these early times, addressing and meeting the country's food sanitation needs seemed like an arduous task. It would be many years before we were to have such luxuries as refrigeration, understand the importance of sanitary food processing standards, and implement good manufacturing processes (GMP). So in many respects, a watchdog agency was necessary. The FDA was, at first, pointed in the right direction. This can be seen clearly in their mission statement, which reads:

"The FDA's mission is to promote and protect the public health by helping safe and effective products reach the market in a timely way, and monitoring products for continued safety after they are in use. Our work is a blending of law and science aimed at protecting consumers."[6]

In its infancy, the FDA can be applauded for introducing foundational science and sanitation issues to the public. For instance, in 1913, the meat packing industry was described as nauseating.[7] To remedy this, the FDA implemented a meat inspection law and a comprehensive food and drug law. This made it possible for producers to bring safer food items to market. Ultimately, this provided better health to the American public and was completely in line with their mission statement.

In order to protect consumers from dangerous products in other markets, the FDA expanded its reach by enhancing the Pure Food and Drug Act of 1906 with the 1938 Food, Drug, and Cosmetic Act. This act brought cosmetics and medical devices under direct control of the FDA. It also required pharmaceutical drugs to be labeled with adequate directions for safe use. But most notably, it required pre-market approval of all new, man-made drugs.

By passing the 1938 Food, Drug, and Cosmetic Act into law, the FDA was given an unprecedented, broad jurisdiction over all food, drugs and medical devices. Because of this legislation, the FDA has had sole power in determining which foods, drugs and medical devices have made it to the marketplace since 1938. The FDA also determines how these products will be labeled, used and marketed. Combined with its mission statement, this wide range of authority gave birth to

---

[6]   http://www.fda.gov.

[7]   *As described in* Upton Sinclair's novel, *The Jungle.*

the myth that FDA approved drugs are safe and effective. As a result, thousands of FDA approved drugs are prescribed and consumed every day. Most people not only trust that they are safe, but also consider them a "god-send." Aside from use in emergency medicine, research findings on many commonly used prescription drugs quickly expose this health myth.

A good example of this is the FDA approved drug known as Posicor (a chemical called mibefradil dihydrochloride). Posicor was approved in 1997 for the treatment of high blood pressure (hypertension). Prior to approval, the data from the congestive heart failure trials presented at a FDA Advisory Committee meeting on Posicor showed that more patients treated with Posicor died than those taking a placebo.

This did not stop the FDA's approval of Posicor. After its release for use by the public, 200 more Americans died from using Posicor as prescribed. It was finally removed from the market in 1998.[8] Not surprisingly, and despite the known dangers and real-life data, the drug manufacturer Hoffman-La Roche Inc. insisted that "Mibefradil [Posicor] proved a safe, well-tolerated, and effective antianginal agent that can be used regardless of demographic factors or of frequently coexisting clinical conditions."[9]

Both the dangers of prescription drugs and the greed of the pharmaceutical industry are glaringly obvious when we study the FDA approved drug Prozac (fluoxetine). Fluoxetine is one of the most commonly prescribed anti-depressant medications to date. The popularity of Prozac is a result of marketing, not science. In 1990, Prozac appeared on the cover of *Newsweek*

---

[8]   *Journal of the American Medical Association.* Dec 22/29 1999 - Vol. 282, No. 24.

[9]   Charlon V, Kobrin I. "The efficacy and safety of mibefradil in subgroups of patients with chronic stable angina pectoris." *International Journal of Clinical Practice.* 1998 Jun; 52(4): 257-64.

magazine with the headline "Prozac: A Breakthrough Drug for Depression."[10]

Looking at the history behind Prozac not only shows the grip that the pharmaceutical industry has on the media, but also the much darker side of this commonly prescribed antidepressant. Scientists at Eli Lilly developed Prozac in the 1970's. It was believed that this drug could selectively inhibit the reuptake of serotonin (a brain neurotransmitter that has been shown to alter mood and behavior) and so could be used to treat depression. The first testing of Prozac was performed on dogs and cats. Every trial showed that Prozac use caused aggression amongst these normally calm and friendly animals, as could be seen by increased hissing and growling. When the animals were taken off of the drug, they returned to their usual friendly behavior. This testing concluded that Prozac use causes aggressive behavior.

By mid 1978, Prozac testing moved to humans in controlled clinical trials, where over 4000 patients were involved. In an attempt to obtain positive evidence of its safety and effectiveness, the study allowed for voluntary dropout of those who experienced the most severe side effects. Additionally, clinical investigators were allowed to administer concurrent sedatives to patients to mask the side effects that would most likely to lead to violence/suicide. Thus, many of the negative side effects were not reported due to dropouts or masking from sedatives. Despite the lack of scientific methodology, this study concluded that Prozac works well to a "statistically significant" degree in a population of depressed patients.

Both of these animal and human studies raised red flags about a potential causal relationship between Prozac and vio-

---

[10] Hegerty, James. *Suicidal and violent behavior with the use of fluoxetine.* 1995. See www.hsph.harvard.edu/Organizations/DDIL/prozac.html.

lence/suicide. Furthermore, Eli Lilly did not then, nor do they now, know how or why fluoxetine controls behavior. Consequently, Eli Lilly and medical doctors have no way of knowing how Prozac elevates the mood of some individuals, nor do they know how any individual will respond emotionally or physically to the drug. Despite these alarming truths, Eli Lilly obtained FDA approval in 1987 and launched drug sales in early 1988 by labeling Prozac a selective serotonin reuptake inhibitor (SSRI).

Since its approval, the potential for Prozac-induced suicide has become frighteningly clear amongst both professionals and the public. Reports of Prozac-associated suicide, written by James D. Hagerty and distributed by the Drugs and Devices Information Line at the Harvard School of Public Health, dominated the Letters to the Editor section of the *American Journal of Psychiatry* during the fall of 1990.[11] Under the FDA's own analysis, there have been more than 20,000 Prozac-related suicides since 1987. Clinical studies performed on Prozac show 191 negative side effects per 100 people.[12] This equates to almost two negative side effects for every user of the drug.

The greed behind the creators of Prozac knows no end. Despite the many adverse side effects associated with it, the FDA approved its use for children in 2003! To make matters even worse, the FDA granted its manufacturer, Eli Lilly, extended patent protection. In order to procure 30 additional months of earning power, Eli Lilly changed the name of Prozac to Sarafem, while at the same time labeling a normal

[11] Hegarty, James, D. "Suicidal and violent behavior associated with the use of fluoxetine." *Drugs and Devices Information Line at the Harvard School of Public Health.* Copyright 1995. www.hsph.harvard.edu/Organizations/DDIL/prozac.html

[12] Cohen, S. Jay. Over Dose. 2001. ISBN 1-58542-123-5.

Prozac

occurrence among women a disease; this "disease" being premenstrual irritability. As a result, thousands of unsuspecting women were given Prozac for premenstrual irritability while at the same time increasing their chances of suffering from the aforementioned negative side effects such as violence, aggression, and suicide.

With respect to controlling mood, L-tryptophan is superior to commonly prescribed antidepressants such as Prozac and other SSRI's. This fact is due to the mechanism by which L-tryptophan works in the body. Unlike SSRI's, L-tryptophan helps the body produce more serotonin by serving as a "building block" of this amino acid. Conversely, prescription drugs work to elongate the actions of naturally occurring serotonin. Herein lies the problem. If an individual is not actively producing serotonin, for whatever reason, then the prescription drug is useless and begins to elicit numerous negative side effects. Additionally, problems with mood and appetite control can continue or even worsen. Using L-tryptophan, users will have plenty of serotonin, which will result in numerous benefits associated with the activity of serotonin such as enhanced mood, appetite control and good sleep.

Prozac is not Eli Lilly's only problem child. Their highly touted antipsychotic, Zyprexa, is yet another example of FDA approved drugs being unsafe and ineffective. Clinical trials lasting a mere six weeks showed that the drug was linked to life-threatening side effects requiring hospitalization in 22% of those treated. A weight gain of 50-70 pounds was common among users. Worse yet, studies showed that users were 10 times more likely to suffer from Type-II Diabetes as a result of taking the drug even short term! During the 6-week clinical trials for Zyprexa there were 20 deaths. Among these deaths,

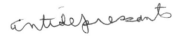

antidepressants

12 were suicides.[13] Dr. David Healy has stated that clinical trials surrounding Zyprexa "Demonstrate a higher death rate on Zyprexa than on any other antipsychotic ever recorded." The *Baltimore Sun* has stated that the FDA has done little to warn doctors and consumers.[14] Eli Lilly advertises at www.zyprexa.com the following with respect to Zyprexa: "Helping You Get Better."

The FDA's trend to blatantly disregard the public's health continues even with the FDA approved vaccines given to our children. On October 22, 1999, The Advisory Committee on Immunization Practices (ACIP) decided that Rotashield, the only US-licensed rotavirus vaccine (for infant diarrhea), should no longer be recommended for infants in the United States. This recommendation was based on the fact that over 100 babies within the first year of approval suffered from obstructed bowels as a direct result of the vaccine. This painful condition is known as intussusception and treatment usually involves surgery.

The public was led to believe that this negative side effect was newly discovered. To the contrary, on June 15, 2000, the Committee on Government Reform reported that it was well known during clinical trials and the licensing process that there were increased incidences of obstructed bowels amongst newly-vaccinated babies. vaccines

It would appear that it was neither safety nor effectiveness that enabled the Rotashield vaccine to acquire FDA approval, but rather vested financial interests at the FDA. Of those participating in the Rotashield approval meeting, over half of the voters had financial ties to the Rotashield vaccine. Such ties

---

[13]   Sharav, Vera Hassner. *14th Tri-Service Clinical Investigation Symposium. May 5-7, 2002.*

[14]   "Studies Link Zyprexa to Diabetes & Deaths." *Baltimore Sun.* See http://www.ahrp.org/infomail/0303/20.html.

included being paid as consultants, lobbyists, owning stock in the company, holding vaccine patents, or being employed by institutions or companies who would benefit from the Rotashield vaccine approval. While this practice is forbidden, waivers were conveniently granted by the Centers for Disease Control (CDC)![15] Other commonly administered FDA approved vaccines also show dangers associated with them.

The New England Journal of Medicine reported that the MMR vaccine is responsible for 35% of juvenile rheumatoid arthritis cases. An analysis of the Adverse Events Reporting System (AERS) database from 1991 through 1998 showed that the rubella vaccine caused 55% of females vaccinated to develop rheumatoid arthritis.

With regards to the DPT vaccine, Roger R. Gervais, BSc, DC, ND, reports that "One in every 100 children react with convulsions or collapse or high-pitched screaming to the DTP vaccine. One out of every three of these – that is one out of every 300 – will remain permanently damaged."

Testimony of the former Assistant Secretary of Health, Edward Grant, Jr, before the United States Senate Committee on May 3, 1985, stated "every year, 35,000 children suffer neurological damage because of the DTP vaccine."

Further evidence regarding the pertussis vaccine (for whooping cough), also known as DTP, shows that babies die at a rate of seven times greater than normal within three days after receiving the vaccine. This phenomenon is egregiously disguised as SIDS. The *Journal of Pediatrics* has informed us that the pertussis vaccine is only 40-45% effective and yet this is not sustained. During a pertussis outbreak in Ohio, 82%

---

[15]   Majority Staff Report. Committee on Government Reform. US House of Representatives. June 15th, 2000. *Conflicts of Interest in Vaccine Making Policy.*

of those children who suffered from it were vaccinated! Many more vaccine facts can be found in Neil Miller's book entitled *Vaccines, Are they Really Safe and Effective?*

The profit motives behind vaccines, while blatantly clear from the rotavirus vaccine, can also be seen by the fact that parents are falsely made to believe that their children are required to have them in order to attend public schools. This is a FALLACY steeped in profit motives. All state laws assert that your child is EXEMPT from receiving vaccinations if you have a religious conviction or personal belief opposed to vaccinations.

In addition to vaccines, the health of our children is also threatened by the FDA approved drug Ritalin (methylphenidate). The Experimental Pharmacology Department of the American Cyanamid Company and the Merck Index reports that Ritalin is no less toxic or safer than amphetamine and methamphetamine. They continue by stating that with the administration of this drug, motor activity decreases. Many times, tremors and convulsions occur. Studies on amphetamine derivatives show that short-term clinical doses produce brain cell death. Long-lasting and sometimes permanent changes in the biochemistry of the brain are also a result.

The Drug Enforcement Administration (DEA) classifies *Ritalin*
Ritalin, as well as Dexedrine (dextroamphetamine), Desoxyn (methamphetamine), and Adderral (a mixture of Ritalin, Dexedrine, and amphetamine) in the same Schedule II category as methamphetamine and cocaine. Both methamphetamine and cocaine are targeted by the "war on drugs." This did not stop FDA approval of Ritalin and an entire class of stimulants for use in children.

Paradoxically, while parents and doctors are relentlessly feeding their children "approved" stimulant drugs that match the lethality of methamphetamine and cocaine; the United

States Government spends nearly $1 billion dollars per month to fight the war on drugs. One weapon in this war is the D.A.R.E. Program. D.A.R.E. is taught by police officers who put people in jail for using "crank" and "speed." Yet, while learning "Drug Abuse Resistance" through D.A.R.E., it seems that 60% of the "attendees" are intoxicated and debilitated by these street drugs known as "crank" or "speed."

Currently, the FDA approved drug. (bupropion), AKA Zyban, is being heavily marketed as a weight-loss pill. The July 2003 issue of *Obesity Research* reported that subjects who completed 26 weeks of bupropion use maintained mean losses of 4.6% of baseline weight for those taking bupropion (SR 300 mg/dL) while those on placebo lost 1.8% of baseline weight.[16, 17] This equates to a "whopping" 2.8% loss in body weight.

But is it really "whopping"? A 2.8% loss in body weight is equivalent to a 200 pound woman who is 5'8" tall losing 5.6 pounds. This would bring her weight to 195 pounds. Using a more accurate figure for beneficial weight loss, her BMI would have gone from 30 (classifying her as scientifically obese) to 30! Thus, Wellbutrin, scientifically and factually, has zero benefit for weight loss!

Nonetheless, experts for weight loss often tout this FDA approved drug while the side effects are typically not discussed. For example, Dr. Richard Atkinson, president of the American Obesity Association, has declared that, "This is a drug that people have taken for many years to treat depression with few problems or side effects."

Unfortunately, clinical studies show otherwise. Looking at the actions of the drug, *Clinical Pharmacology* gave what seems

---

[16] *Obesity Research.* 2002 Jul;10 (7):633-641. *Obesity Research.* 2002 Oct;10 (10):1049-56.

[17] Lipman, Larry. *Health Policy Journal Health Affairs.* July 9th, 2002.

to be a warning rather than a mechanism of action. "Bupropion is a novel antidepressant whose mechanism of action must still be elucidated."[18] And further, "The mechanism of action of the novel antidepressant bupropion remains unclear after many years of study."

The *Journal of Clinical Psychology* asserts, "Bupropion is widely distributed to tissues and extensively metabolized by oxidation and reduction to at least six metabolites, some of which may be active. Bupropion does not inhibit monoamine oxidase, exerts no effect on serotonin uptake, and minimally alters the reuptake of norepinephrine at presynaptic sites. It does not appear to exert action leading to postsynaptic beta-adrenergic down-regulation, and it has minimal inhibitory effects on presynaptic dopamine uptake."[19] In other words, bupropion does not display any of the mechanisms of action that would be expected in an antidepressant. If it's not an antidepressant, then what is it, and why has it been approved as such?

Wellbutrin was pulled off the market in 1986 because of an unacceptable incidence of seizures. The FDA released it back to the market later that year for unknown reasons. According to clinical trials, 6.1% of users will suffer from withdrawals due to adverse events from using the drug. Additionally, it is well known that all Wellbutrin-related seizures occurred in patients who are taking what is considered to be a therapeutic dose of 450 mg/day or less. However, real-life data is suggesting much higher rates of adverse reactions. Wellbutrin is the third leading cause of drug related seizures with cocaine being number one.[20] Health Canada and GlaxoSmithKline (the same company who funded the aforementioned weight loss study)

[18]   Clinical Pharmacology 1983 Nov-Dec;2 (6):525-37.
[19]   *Journal of Clinical Psychiatry.* 1983 May; 44 (5 Pt 2): 74-8.
[20]   *Journal of Emergency Medicine.* 2002 Apr; 22 (3): 235-9 J.

received 1,127 reports of adverse reactions to Wellbutrin between May 1998 and May 28, 2001. Among these were 19 deaths and 172 reports of seizures or convulsions. To make matters worse, the Medicines Control Agency (equivalent to FDA) of Britain has confirmed 18 deaths and received reports of 3,457 patients complaining of adverse reactions from 2000-2001. Despite these staggering figures, the number of children being prescribed Wellbutrin jumped 195% between 1995 and 1999.[21] Somebody should be tried and convicted.

On June 26, 2003, GlaxoSmithKline, manufacturer of Wellbutrin, announced that it had received an approval letter from the FDA for an extended-release formulation of its widely used antidepressant Wellbutrin.

Heart patients beware: While millions take medication to prevent heart problems, it appears that antiarrhythmia drugs are more dangerous than a failing heart. Two FDA approved antiarrhythmia (for treatment of irregular heart beat) drugs known as flecainide and encainide clearly suppress arrhythmias. Unfortunately, studies also show that they also suppress the heartbeat in general, proved by the fact that 2.5 times as many patients taking these drugs die as opposed to those that do not take these drugs![22]

By far, the FDA approved cholesterol-lowering drugs deserve the most attention. While most Americans have developed a love affair for these drugs, very few are aware of their negative side effects. Unknown to the public and most doc-

---

[21] *Journal of the American Medical Association.* April 17, 2002 - Vol. 287, No. 15.

[22] Kauffman, Joel. "Should You Take Aspirin to Prevent Heart Attack?" *Journal of Scientific Exploration.* Vol. 14, No. 4, pp.623-641, 2000; and "Special report: Preliminary report: Effect of encainide and flecainide on mortality in a randomized trial of arrhythmia suppression after myocardial infarction." *New England Journal of Medicine.* 1989; 321: 406-412. [No authors listed].

tors, cholesterol lowering drugs can be life threatening.[23] In a letter to the *Archives of Internal Medicine*, Uffe Ravnskov, MD, PhD and colleagues show that in two of the three clinical trials that included healthy people, the chance of survival was better without the use of cholesterol lowering drugs.[24] Numerous medical journals have shown that cholesterol-lowering drugs significantly increase one's risk of suffering from CoQ10 deficiency (paradoxically, low CoQ10 is associated with congestive heart failure), rhabdomyolysis (muscle deterioration causing pain and weakness), kidney failure, erectile dysfunction, loss of memory (transient global amnesia) and loss of mental focus.

In conclusion, the previously mentioned drugs are not isolated incidents of FDA negligence and deceit. The list of FDA approved drugs that are unsafe and ineffective goes on. To find this list we don't have to look far. It's already been compiled in the Physicians Desk Reference (PDR). A random journey through the PDR would show that the majority of FDA approved drugs are toxic with very little benefit.

Why does the FDA have a history of approving deadly drugs? This is the first question that comes to mind when learning of the atrocities caused by medications that carry the FDA label. A bit of investigation into who controls the FDA offers great insight as to why FDA approved drugs are deadly.

According to USA Today, over half of the experts hired by the FDA to advise the government on the safety and effectiveness of medicines have direct financial relationships with the pharmaceutical companies who will either be helped or hurt by the decision of FDA approval. These conflicts include helping a pharmaceutical company invent a medicine, then serving

---

[23]   Cohen, S. Jay. *Over Dose*. 2001. ISBN 1-58542-123-5.
[24]   Uffe Ravnskov, et al. *Letter to Archives of Internal Medicine*, submitted on July 20, 2002.

on the FDA advisory committee, which then decides whether or not the drug will be approved for human consumption. Most of the time, conflicts are in the form of stock ownership and obtaining consulting fees or research grants from the drug industry.

A USA TODAY analysis of financial conflicts of interest from Jan 1, 1998 to June 30, 1999 shows the following, based on 159 FDA advisory committee meetings:

- 92% of the meetings had at least one member who had a financial conflict of interest

- At 55% of advisory meetings, at least half, sometimes more of the FDA advisers had conflicts of interest

- Financial conflicts of interest were most frequent at the 57 meetings when broader issues were discussed: 92% of members had conflicts

- At 102 meetings dealing with the fate of a given drug, 33% of the experts in attendance had a financial conflict

Historically, the FDA had revealed when these financial conflicts were present, but these conflicts have been kept secret since 1992.[25] Hence, it is impossible to determine the amounts of money or the pharmaceutical companies involved. Worse yet, federal law prohibits the FDA from using experts with financial conflicts of interest to decide whether or not certain medications should be approved. However, as pointed out by Jay S. Cohen, MD, the FDA has waived this restriction 800 times since 1998![26]

---

[25] Cauchon, Dennis. *USA Today*. 09/25/00.

[26] Cohen, JS. *Over Dose: The Case Against The Drug Companies. Prescription Drugs, Side Effects, and Your Health.* Tarcher/Putnam, New York: October 2001.

The pharmaceutical companies' grip on the FDA is the primary reason that deadly and ineffective drugs are approved. Understanding this allows us to better understand the importance of thinking twice before "following doctor's orders." More specifically, pharmaceutical campaigning led to the passage of the 1997 Food and Drug Administration Modernization Act (FDAMA). The FDAMA allows for a new drug's approval based on only one clinical trial.

As we have seen from the above examples, lowering drug approval standards is having and continues to have horrendous consequences to the health of Americans. Between 1997 and 2001 a total of 12 commonly prescribed FDA approved drugs were removed from the market only after serious side effects, or in some cases after hundreds of injuries and deaths, occurred.[27] These drugs included Pondimin, Redux, Seldane, Posicor, Duracht, Hismanal, Raxar, Rezulin, Propulsid, Lotronex, Raplon, and Baycol.

Profiting from other people's pain is GREAT business. Despite their lack of safety and effectiveness, the aforementioned drugs generated $5 billion dollars in sales for the pharmaceutical giants! Not surprisingly, the FDAMA remains intact and a drug company can still gain approval based on ONE clinical trial.

The pharmaceutical companies' grip on the FDA has squeezed out even more benefits for the drug industry. In addition to lowering drug approval standards, pharmaceutical companies have ensured that the FDA is well compensated for their approval. Once again, pharmaceutical campaigning led to the Prescription Drug User Fee Act (PDUFA) of 1992 and it's reauthorization in 1997. The PDUFA allows the FDA to collect fees from pharmaceutical companies to review

---

[27]   Copyright © 2003 PBSI and wgbh/frontline.

FDA *primary source for pharmaceutical industry*

new drug applications. This sets a new precedent in drug approval. Previously, the United States treasury funded the FDA. However, with the PDUFA, they now receive their paychecks directly from the pharmaceutical industry. Hence, while the FDA once regulated drug approval, granting that approval is now a moneymaker for the FDA. This ensures that the FDA remains the prime source of drug dealing for the pharmaceutical industry.

Sidney Wolfe, MD, Director of Public Citizen's Health Research Group since its founding in 1971, has summed up the end result of the pharmaceutical grip on the FDA by stating that the culture at the FDA has become, "Please the industry. Avoid conflict. Look upon our role as getting out as many drugs as possible."

Congressman Dan Burton has recognized this deadly trend among the FDA as well. In a noble attempt to notify other members of congress he has testified the following:

"How confident can we be in the recommendations with the Food and Drug Administration when the chairman [of Vaccines and Related Biological Products Advisory Committee] and other individuals on their advisory committee own stock in major manufacturers of vaccines? How confident can we be in a system when the agency seems to feel that the number of experts is so few that everyone has a conflict and thus waivers must be granted? It almost appears that there is an "old boys' network" of vaccine advisors that rotate between the CDC and FDA—at times serving both simultaneously...It is important to determine if the Department of Health and Human Services has become complacent in their implementation of the legal requirements on conflicts of interest and committee management. If the law is too loose, we need to change it. If the agencies aren't doing their job, they need to be held

Vaccines stock

accountable ... What is at issue is not whether researchers can be bought in the sense of a quid pro quo, it is that close and remunerative collaboration with a company naturally creates goodwill on the part of researchers and the hope that the largesse will continue...Can the FDA and the CDC really believe that scientists are more immune to self-interest than other people?"[28]

Learning more about the pharmaceutical grip from key experts, we look to Michael Elashoff, an ex-FDA biostatistician, who has stated that, "The people in charge [FDA officials] don't say 'Should we approve this drug?' They say 'Hey, how can we get this drug approved?'"[29]

Conflicts of interest within the FDA by the pharmaceutical community have been clearly illustrated in some of the most well respected medical journals. The *British Medical Journal* has published the comments of Paul Stolley, MD, MPH, a former senior consultant to the FDA. He says "The agency [the FDA] neglects drug safety in its rush to speed the drug-approval process because current laws and policies let the drug industry influence FDA decisions."[30]

Dr. William L. Isley of Kansas City, MO, sheds more light on the situation by stating, "The FDA used to serve a purpose. A doctor could feel sure that the drug he was prescribing was as safe as possible. Now you wonder what kind of evaluation has been done, and what's been swept under the rug." Thus,

---

[28] Glode, Elizabeth R. "Advising Under the Influence? Conflicts of Interest Among FDA Advisory Committee Members." Copyright © 2002. *The Food and Drug Law Institute Food and Drug Law Journal.* 2002. 57;293.

[29] Willman, David. "How a New Policy Led to Seven Deadly Drugs." *Los Angeles Times.* December 20, 2000.

[30] DeNoon, Daniel. "Drug Safety Not FDA Priority." *WebMD.* Sept 12, 2002.

Shane Ellison M.Sc. *doctors*

without a strong understanding of organic chemistry, physiology, and biochemistry it has become virtually impossible for the average medical doctor to obtain straightforward, non-biased data surrounding synthetic medicines.

The conflict of interest amongst the FDA has become so apparent that it has caught the attention of major university researchers. A team of Harvard University professors has publicly advised physicians NOT to prescribe new drugs to their patients because their safety has not been established, despite FDA approval! To support this warning, the professors acknowledged that adverse drug reactions (ADRs) from FDA approved drugs are the leading cause of death in America.[31]

Call it human nature, greed, or just plain old corruption; the protective mechanism that was once the driving force of the FDA is gone. Over the years it has been taken over by international pharmaceutical companies who make every effort to push the "FDA approval" on unsuspecting American victims. The FDA has a myriad of "skeletons in the closet" and has repeatedly shown blatant disregard for the public's health while enriching their pharmaceutical partners. According to the actions of the FDA, an insidious and out-of-control foreigner has moved in and become the self-proclaimed watchdog under the guise of the FDA.

Undoubtedly, prior to the advent of this book, America has been grossly ignorant of the FDA's deadly bias for wealth not health. As pharmaceutical business has grown, the FDA has changed from an institution that was trying to protect public health from bad food to a rubber stamp government organization that only takes public health into account when it is forced to by some form of gross public error.

31   Lasser KE; et al. "Timing of New Black Box Warnings and Withdrawals for Prescription Medications." *Journal of the American Medical Association.* May 1, 2002, 287:2215-2220.

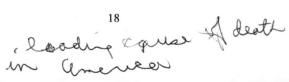
leading cause of death in America

To procure a lifetime of health, Americans will have to accept the dark side of health freedom by taking responsibility for their own lives and well being rather than depending on the FDA to protect them.

Myth #2 - Drug Advertising Promotes Health Awareness for Consumers

Fact: Drug companies are often allowed to get away with false advertising, which they use to "educate" both the public and doctors about their products in order to increase sales!

Do you feel safe knowing that these misleading advertisements are frequently the *only* source of education for your doctor on the drugs that he prescribes for your family? *no*

Despite guidelines set by the FDA, pharmaceutical companies are often in violation of the Federal Food, Drug and Cosmetic Act (FFDCA) by making false and misleading claims about their drugs in advertisements. This false and misleading advertising to both patients and medical doctors results in the use of drugs that are far more dangerous and/or less effective than the pharmaceutical industry would like you to believe. This blatant irresponsibility leads to an increase of deaths and injuries caused by prescription drugs that would not have occurred had the truth been known.

Currently, America is consuming more prescription drugs than any other country in the world. It is estimated that pre-

[handwritten annotation: americans drug use 50 % world wide]

scription drug use by Americans comprises over 50% of the total prescription drug use worldwide! This prescription drug addiction is the result of Direct-to-Consumer advertising (DTC Advertising). As DTC advertising increases, so do prescription drug sales.[32]

Whether you are reading a magazine, watching television or listening to the radio, it is guaranteed that you'll be bombarded with drug ads. These ads are examples of DTC Advertising. DTC Advertising is still relatively new and has been the responsibility of the FDA since 1962. The 1962 amendments to the Food, Drug, and Cosmetic Act, which charged the Food and Drug Administration (FDA) with regulating pharmaceutical effectiveness in addition to regulating drug safety, also transferred responsibility for prescription drug advertising from the Federal Trade Commission to the FDA.

In a blatant conflict of interest, the FDA granted the duty of DTC advertising to none other than the pharmaceutical companies themselves in 1997. This act proved to be a further acknowledgement of the pharmaceutical industry's grip on the FDA. Officially, this was done as a means of "promoting health awareness among consumers to ensure their health and safety." Of course, this was not done without setting "guidelines." In an attempt to ensure that DTC Advertising is not deceptive, false or misleading; it became regulated under the authority of the Federal Food, Drug and Cosmetic Act (FFDCA).

The content allowed in DTC Advertising by the FDA is typically the drug name and the condition it is intended to treat, as well as a description of the risks and benefits associated with utilizing the drug. The FFDCA irrefutably prohibits the advertising of false therapeutic claims for pharmaceutical

---

[32] Millstein, Lloyd G. "Prescription Drug Advertising: Is it a Driving Force on Drug Pricing?" *North Carolina Medical Journal.* November/December 2003, Volume 64, Number 6.

drugs and states that the product claim advertisements must meet the following criteria:

- Claims cannot be false or misleading

- Ads must present a fair balance between the risks and benefits of a drug

- Ads must reveal the consequences of using the drug as advertised

- Ads must disclose all the risks listed in the drug's labeling

Hypothetically, DTC advertising *could* have positive effects on health care. As long as consumers are given pertinent information about prescription drugs, they are very capable of making positive health decisions. This strengthens the doctor-patient relationship by ensuring that they can make mutual decisions about drug treatment rather than having the doctor dictate to the patient what is needed. But these goals are only achieved if DTC advertising is honest.

Despite the guidelines, it has been well established that since at least 1997, pharmaceutical companies have engaged in deceitful marketing by:

- Overstating benefits

- Not including data of therapeutic benefits

- Not showing data from clinical trial results and

- Giving an imbalanced view of the benefits and risks of the drug

Worse yet, unscrupulous drug makers have used DTC Advertising as a means of increasing drug sales by promoting prescription drugs as necessary for healthy people. Many bla-

statins, Lipitor

tant examples of false adverting exist among some of the most widely prescribed drugs.

The cholesterol-lowering drugs known as "statins" serve as the best example of deceitful drug marketing. With heavy ad campaigns to promote them and "preferential citation" of supporting clinical trials, which were often sponsored by the drug makers themselves, statins were the most widely sold pharmaceutical drug in 2002.

Specifically, Pfizer has shown blatant disregard for FFDCA criteria when marketing their statin drug Lipitor. They advertise that rhabdomyolysis (i.e. muscle deterioration exhibited by muscle pain, tenderness, or weakness) and myopathy (muscular dystrophies) only occur with "other drugs" in the statin class, not Lipitor (see ads in *Time, Reader's Digest, Good Housekeeping, Woman's Day* and *Health*). As a result, millions of medical doctors regurgitate this claim to their patients in an effort to ensure that they consume Lipitor.

That Lipitor does not elicit rhabdomyolysis was simply a marketing ploy to gain an edge over competing statin drugs. The FDA sent a letter to Pfizer stating that, based on Pfizer's own clinical trials, this was simply untrue. In their letter to Pfizer, the FDA stated that Pfizer's advertisements "fail to disclose that Lipitor has the same potential risk of rhabdomyolysis and myopathy as other lipid-lowering statin drugs." Consequently, they were in clear violation of the FFDCA by making these false claims. Despite Pfizer's non-compliance with the law, the FDA did not press charges.

An interesting point, Pfizer's false advertising isn't the only action taken to procure profits from the sale of Lipitor. Clinical trials showed that Lipitor is effective at doses ranging from 2.5 mg to 5 mg. But Pfizer demands that Lipitor be prescribed starting at 10 mg.[33] This starting dose is approximately 300% higher than the effective dose! Even more astounding, doctors are now prescribing up to 80 mgs of Lipitor!

If you are currently taking statins, this fact explains why you are required to go in for regular liver testing: you are being overdosed! Fortunately, 50% of those who take cholesterol-lowering drugs quit voluntarily due to the negative side effects experienced with this drug.

The statin wars continue in the media with the consumer being the victim. In an attempt to procure a larger market, Lipitor's chemical cousin, Pravachol, is also guilty of false advertising. Made by Bristol Myer Squib, Pravachol is also a statin drug. It is prescribed to patients who do not have coronary heart disease (CHD), but who have high cholesterol and want to prevent heart-related events. In an attempt to reach more users, Bristol Myer Squib used promotional material to broaden the conditions and patient populations for which Pravachol is indicated.

Specifically, the advertisements implied that Pravachol is approved for the prevention of stroke in patients who do not have CHD. The truth be told, Pravachol is only approved for the use of reducing the risk of stroke in patients who have clinical evidence of CHD. Thus, if you do not have CHD then Pravachol is not approved for your use. Ignoring this completely, Bristol Myer Squib profited by marketing Pravachol to healthy people for whom this drug was never approved. Bristol Myer Squib brazenly used DTC advertising to simply invent reasons why YOU need their drug rather than to educate consumers! In a warning letter to Bristol Myer Squib, the FDA makes it clear that DTC advertising of Pravachol went beyond

---

[33]   Cohen, S. Jay. *Over Dose*. 2001. ISBN 1-58542-123-5.

no less deaths from heart disease [handwritten annotation]

the product's approved indications, overstated its effectiveness, and made unsubstantiated effectiveness claims!

While the advertising rhetoric behind statin drugs hints that these drugs help prevent cardiovascular disease (CVD), or more specifically heart disease, the absolute number of deaths from cardiovascular disease – 750,000 deaths per year – has not changed for the last 25 years. In fact, death rates from heart failure, one of the major causes of cardiovascular disease, have doubled since 1986 despite the popularity of cholesterol-lowering drug use![34] Thus, statin drugs are being marketed without showing any quantitative data surrounding their purported therapeutic benefits; which, coincidentally, have NEVER shown to prevent early death from heart disease. More details on this subject will be found in chapter 4.

Of course, false advertising is not endemic to cholesterol-lowering drugs. Purveyors of Hormone Replacement Therapy (HRT) drugs are guilty of false advertising as well. The makers of the Climera brand transdermal estradiol patch, Berlex Laboratories, falsely marketed their HRT drug with the headlines:

"Transdermal ERT – Recommended for the millions of patients with hypertension, hypertriglyceridemia, or gallstones."

The division of Drug Marketing, Advertising and Communications (DDMAC) of the FDA sent a letter to Berlex stating that they were in clear violation of the FFDCA and its implementing regulations. Their violation: Blatant disregard

---

[34] Patrick, Lyn and Uzick, Michael. "Cardiovascular Disease: C-Reactive Protein and the Inflammatory Disease Paradigm: HMG-CoA Reductase Inhibitors, Alpha-Tocopherol, Red Yeast Rice, and Olive Oil Polyphenols. A Review of the Literature." *Alternative Medicine Review*. Volume 6, Number 3. 2001.

of the facts and lying to the public. As pointed out by the FDA, the HRT drug Climera has never been demonstrated to be useful for patients with hypertension, hypertriglyceridemia, or gallstones. Further, while the ads for Climera made false claims about its potential efficacy for preventing hypertension, hypertriglyceridemia, or gallstones, it also failed to disclose the potential negative side effects of HRT.

Berlex is not the only company to disseminate false advertising for HRT. When writing about HRT, the *New York Times* ran articles with the headlines "New Therapy [HRT] Builds Bone without Unpleasant Side Effects." [35] Taking the lies even further, the *Associated Press* promised the world, "Hormones May Lower Risk of Breast Cancer's Return." [36]

A very quick look through the scientific literature regarding the side effects of HRT reveals a number of very disturbing trends. The *Journal of the American Medical Association* (*JAMA*) reported, "Our data adds to the growing body of evidence that recent long-term use of HRT is associated with an increased risk of breast cancer and that such use may be related particularly to lobular tumors." [37]

To add insult to injury, *JAMA* also showed that users of the HRT drug Prempro (combination of estrogen and progestin) develop Alzheimer's at twice the rate of those taking a

---

[35] Zuckerman, D. "Hype in health reporting: "Checkbook science" buys distortion of medical news." *International Journal of Health Services.* 2003;33(2):383-9.

[36] Zuckerman, D. " Hype in health reporting: "Checkbook science" buys distortion of medical news." *International Journal of Health Services.* 2003;33(2):383-9.

[37] Chen CL, Weiss NS, Newcomb P, Barlow W, White E. "Hormone replacement therapy in relation to breast cancer." *Journal of the American Medical Association.* 2002 Feb 13;287(6):734-41.

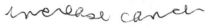

placebo.[38] The *British Medical Journal* recently confirmed the above findings in their most recent issue by stating "long term use of combined HRT doubles cancer risk." [39]

The fact that estrogen and its derivatives increase the incidence of cancer is no surprise. As early as the 1970's, scientists such as Dr. Otto Sartorius, Director of the Cancer Control Clinic, have emphatically made public announcements stating, "Estrogen [and its derivatives] is the fodder on which cancer grows." [40]

Why is HRT labeled as a panacea for all women over the age of 50? Interestingly, it began with Dr. Robert Wilson's book entitled, "Forever Feminine." In it, Dr. Wilson promoted hormones as a miracle cure for "dull and unattractive" women. Once the truth about HRT therapy came to surface, it was discovered that Dr. Wilson's book and its marketing was paid for by Wyeth, a leading distributor of HRT drugs.[41] Sadly, rather than becoming "forever feminine," thousands of women have increased their chances of suffering from cancer, Alzheimer's, and obesity. Meanwhile, drug companies pocketed billions, and still do, from sales of HRT drugs.

The fact that methamphetamine is a highly addictive and dangerous Schedule II drug in the United States has not stopped pharmaceutical companies from dealing this drug via false advertising. Adderall is a cocktail of amphetamine salts,

---

[38] "Estrogen Plus Progestin and the Incidence of Dementia and Mild Cognitive Impairment in Postmenopausal Women." *Journal of the American Medical Association.* 2003;289:2651-2662.

[39] Spurgeon, D. "Long Term use of HRT Doubles Cancer Risk." *British Medical Journal.* 2003 Jul 5;327(7405):9.

[40] 4. Griffin, Edward, G. *World Without Cancer.* ISBN. 0-912986-19-0. American Media.

[41] Zuckerman, D. "Hype in health reporting: "Checkbook science" buys distortion of medical news." *International Journal of Health Services.* 2003;33(2):383-9.

and is manufactured by Shire Richwood, Inc. (Shire). On the street, amphetamine salts are known as Meth, poor man's cocaine, crystal meth, ice, glass, and speed.

Shire is the largest "meth lab" in the country, dealing an estimated $345 million worth of this deadly drug every year. According to a warning letter from the FDA, Shire is in violation of the FFDCA for their false marketing of Adderall for several reasons. These include:

- Claims of superiority over Ritalin

- Claims that if Ritalin did not work for you, then Adderall will

- Claims that in addition to using Adderall for ADHD, you can also use it for depression and narcolepsy

- Failure to provide risk information

- Failure to provide sufficient emphasis of the warnings and contraindications of Adderall

Rather than include this life-saving information, Shire falsely advertised Adderall for use by children. According to Shire marketing material, Adderall has a long half-life, and thus, is "perfect" for kids who want to take speed, rather Adderall, before they go to school so to be private in their use! Capitalizing on this, Shire encouraged parents to "Choose convenience – start school this year with ADDERALL!" Shire insisted that that by letting your kids use Adderall, you would "Achieve efficacy and duration of action without compromising safety!"

What Shire does not tell you is that the safety they were speaking of was the result of a study that they conveniently funded. The study data was presented at the Annual Meeting of the American Psychiatric Association. Amazingly, researchers found the following:

"We were quite encouraged to see that, at this stage of the study, not only has Adderall therapy been safe and efficacious, but every patient showed improvement in core symptoms of the condition, with no evidence of an emerging drug tolerance," said presenter and investigator Richard Weisler, MD.

Every patient! Wow! It would seem that Adderall has achieved something that science rarely, if at all, accomplishes...this being that EVERY patient was successful in his or her treatment. Stressing this point, Dr. Weisler continued:

"Every subject has shown ongoing improvement in symptoms at this 10-month point."

Considering that individual variance is anywhere from 40 to 400 times difference, this is a scientific impossibility. And despite the rave review by Shire researchers, the DEA is well aware of the dangers of methamphetamine salts and has conveniently published these dangers on their web site. The dangers include:

- Effects of usage include addiction, psychotic behavior, and brain damage

- Withdrawal symptoms include depression, anxiety, fatigue, paranoia, aggression, and intense cravings

- Chronic use can cause violent behavior, anxiety, confusion, insomnia, auditory hallucinations, mood disturbances, delusions, and paranoia

- Damage to the brain caused by meth usage is similar to Alzheimer's disease, stroke, and epilepsy

To make sure that the DEA is correct in their safety profile of methamphetamine salts, we cross-referenced these facts
with the authoritative Merck Index and The Experimental
Pharmacology Department of the American Cyanamid Company. They report, that upon administration of these drugs
(not after decades of use but upon administration), motor
activity decreases. Frequently, tremors and convulsions occur.
Citing numerous studies on amphetamine salts, they report
that short-term clinical doses produce brain cell death and
that long-lasting and sometimes permanent changes in the
biochemistry of the brain can occur. It would appear that the
DEA is correct.

Nevertheless, medical doctors fell for the false marketing
and Shire-funded research results. As a result, children can
"say no to drugs" and simply ask Mom or Dad to take them
to the doctor's office. According to their web site, Shire insists
that Adderall has "a 60-plus-year history of safety and efficacy." There is no difference, chemically; between the street
drugs we warn our children against and Shire's product.

Shire is not the only company guilty for the false marketing of highly addictive drugs. Purdue Pharma L.P., makers of the highly addictive OxyContin (oxycodone HCl con-
trolled-release), has followed the same path. According to the
FDA, Purdue Pharma L.P. circulated false DTC advertising
through their endorsements of OxyContin in the world's most
prestigious medical journals, most notably the *Journal of the
American Medical Association (JAMA)*. Like so many other
pharmaceutical companies, Purdue Pharma L.P. used DTC
advertising and *JAMA* to promote OxyContin for uses beyond
those for which OxyContin has been proven safe and effective.
Moreover, while promoting OxyContin for obtaining a "Life
with Relief," they failed to publish the potentially fatal risks
associated with the use of this Schedule II substance.

Shane Ellison M.Sc.

Being cited more than once, the FDA warning letters to Michael Friedman, Executive Vice President and Chief Operating Officer of Purdue Pharma L.P., noted that he was in clear violation of FFDCA for making unsubstantiated claims of effectiveness while at the same time "grossly overstating the safety profile" of OxyContin. Considering the well-documented dangers and addictive properties of OxyContin, this is an incorrigible disregard of human life and the laws set by the FFDCA.

False advertising of OxyContin did not cease with the JAMA ads. As part of its marketing and promotion of OxyContin, Purdue Pharma L.P. distributed 15,000 copies of an OxyContin video to physicians without submitting it to the FDA for review. Entitled '*I Got My Life Back: Patients in Pain Tell Their Story,*' presented the pain relief experiences of various patients and the pain medications, including OxyContin, they had been prescribed.

FDA regulations require pharmaceutical manufacturers to submit all promotional materials for approved prescription drug products to the FDA at the time of their initial use. Not surprisingly, Purdue Pharma L.P. did not comply with this regulation. Thus, the FDA did not have an opportunity to review the video to ensure that the information it contained was truthful, balanced, and accurately communicated. Purdue and the FDA acknowledged the oversight of not submitting the video to FDA for approval, yet no action was taken.

Releasing a second version of the video, Purdue Pharma L.P. followed legal procedure by submitting it to the FDA for review. Though, in its report to Congress, the General Accounting Office (GAO) stated that the FDA failed to review the video until after release. Further, it was discovered that, like the first video, it too made unsubstantiated claims and minimized the risks associated with OxyContin. Most astounding, Purdue Pharma L.P. made the unsubstantiated claim that OxyContin had been shown to cause addiction in less than 1 percent of patients! That's a damned lie.

Pushing for approval by the FDA in 1995, Purdue Pharma L.P. insisted that OxyContin be used for cancer pain. Obviously, its uses have grown widely, thanks in part to false DTC advertising. This false marketing led to a huge profit for its maker, Purdue Pharma, who sold $1 billion worth of Oxy-Contin in less than five years.

Thanks to DTC advertising, the truth about OxyContin is unknown among most medical doctors. OxyContin is an opiod agonist, which possesses powerful addictive properties. Consider that the number of people who used OxyContin for illicit purposes at least once increased from 399,000 in 2000 to 957,000 in 2001 according to a recent U.S. Department of Health and Human Services release.[42] These addictive properties are akin to heroin and morphine and know no boundaries of destruction. Its addictive nature can smother even the strongest of wills. Recognizing this, the DEA has listed Oxy-Contin as a Schedule II controlled substance in the USA.

Exactly how OxyContin works in the body is not understood. But its dangers are well documented. OxyContin produces respiratory depression. Additionally, Oxycodone causes a reduction in motility associated with an increase in smooth muscle tone in the antrum of the stomach and duodenum. As a result, digestion of food in the small intestine is delayed or nonexistant, and propulsive contractions are decreased, culminating in constipation and the back up of fecal matter.

According to the DEA, since its release on the market, the annual number of prescriptions for the "synthetic morphine" has risen from around 300,000 to nearly 6 million. During

---

[42]   Health and Human Services press release. September 5, 2002.

OxyContin - constipation

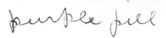

that same period, the number of oxycodone-related deaths has skyrocketed by 400%. Currently, OxyContin is the number-one prescribed Schedule II narcotic in the United States, accounting for 7.7 million prescriptions in 2003.

In a most aggressive attempt to bypass FDA regulations, makers of Nexium should get an award for their creativity. Running drug ads for the "purple pill," Nexium maker Astra-Zeneca skirted all FDA regulations by simply not stating the name of the drug. Instead, they called it the "Healing Purple Pill." Capitalizing on this loophole, their ad failed to describe the condition it is intended to treat, as well as a description of the risks and benefits associated with taking the drug. Overnight, AstraZeneca obtained unbridled marketing power and convinced millions that it was a panacea.

Numerous drug companies have followed this lead. Schering-Plough raked in their share of profits using this marketing technique for Claritin. By stating the drug's name but not what it was used for, the ads for Claritin were exempt from FDA regulations and did not need to disclose the drug's risks or benefits; a clear violation of the FFDCA. As far as the public was concerned, Claritin was the next best thing since Dairy Queen. Millions of people stampeded to the doctor's office for their prescription without knowing the risks or benefits associated with Claritin. This popularity eventually resulted in the approval of Claritin as an OTC drug. Not surprisingly, the four clinical trials showing its safety for OTC use were conveniently performed by Schering-Plough.

Deceitful drug advertising is not limited to the USA. The *Medical Journal of Australia* (*MJA*) has taken note of the false advertising by pointing out the half-truths and shortage of statistics found in DTC advertising by international drug makers. In the *MJA*, authors Newby and Henry present data from the analysis of 174 advertisements for pharmaceuticals. Among these ads designed to "educate the public," fewer than 8% of the advertisements contained quantitative data surrounding the therapeutic benefits of the drug and only 28% published clinical outcomes. In other words, the advertisements failed to disclose how many people benefited from the drug, if any, and whether or not safety and effectiveness was established in a clinical setting.

These are not isolated cases of false advertising among FDA approved drugs. The prevalence of false DTC advertising by drug companies has caught the attention of Blue Cross Blue Shield of America (BCBSA). According to BCBSA's review of DTC advertised drugs, some of the most heavily-promoted drug products have been the target of warning letters or notice of violation letters charging that their DTC advertisements were "False, lacking in fair balance, or otherwise in violation of the Federal Food, Drug, and Cosmetic Act."

As of this writing, FDA commissioner Mark McClellan, MD, PhD, has publicly admitted the faults of DTC advertising in general by stating, "Physicians and others are concerned that consumers may not always get a balanced view of the benefits and risks of a product." [43] Despite the FDA's knowledge of their deceitful advertising, no pharmaceutical company has ever been charged by the FDA for violations of the FFDCA.

Knowing that the false advertisement of prescription drugs can be dangerous and even fatal, the FDA has full power to criminally prosecute violators under the FFDCA. With a flood of multiple warnings to pharmaceutical companies, this is a possibility that must become a reality through vigilant enforcement. Still though, in the context of DTC advertising, the FDA has looked away. For example, a series of 11 illegal ads for Claritin (8 DTC), 14 illegal ads for Flonase/Flovent (8

---

[43]   Elliot, Victoria Stagg, American Medical News Staff, April 28th, 2003.

Shane Ellison M.Sc.

DTC) (Flonase and Flovent are the same drug in two versions, one used for allergy, the other for asthma) and five illegal ads for Celebrex (1 DTC) have been ignored with no criminal actions taken.

The only action taken by the FDA has been letter writing to those companies that have violated the FFDCA. In these letters, the FDA makes it clear that the given pharmaceutical company is in violation of the FFDCA due to overstating benefits, displaying inaccurate safety profiles, and minimizing the risk of side effects.[44] But after that, the FDA remains silent, a paper tiger.

To date, no drug company has ever been charged for their blatant violations of the FFDCA. What is the point of having a regulation if it is not enforced? And how is the FDA protecting consumers if they allow violations of the FFDCA among DTC advertising?

The pharmaceutical industry maintains that DTC advertising is an important vehicle for conveying information to medical doctors.[45] Their stance is not surprising, as DTC Advertising is the Holy Grail for corporate drug pushing. According to the United States General Accounting Office (GAO), sales for DTC-advertised drugs increase 20% faster than sales for drugs that are not heavily advertised to consumers. In their summary, the GAO reported that regardless of their lack of safety and effectiveness, DTC advertising always increases the sale of the given drug. Due to the profit potential and lack of FDA enforcement, DTC advertising is here to

---

[44] Department of Health and Human Services. Food and Drug Administration. Nov. 14, 2000.
Cohen, S. Jay. *Over Dose.* 2001. ISBN 1-58542-123-5.
[45] Henry, David A and Newby, David. "Drug Advertising: Truths, half truths and few statistics." *Medical Journal of Australia.* 2002 177 (6): 285-286.

stay. Currently, pharmaceutical companies are increasing their spending on DTC advertising faster than they are increasing spending on research and development. Drug companies are spending about $2 to $3 billion annually to unleash false advertising campaigns.[46, 47]

With the increase in drug spending due to DTC advertising, we will no doubt see an enormous surge in adverse drug events (ADE's) among those who are not aware of the false and misleading claims behind DTC advertising. Ultimately, this type of advertising, which has become common amongst drug companies, results in prescriptions being written for drugs that are more dangerous and/or less effective than perceived by either doctor or patient. Subsequently, this leads to deaths and injuries that would not have occurred had safer, more effective drugs been prescribed.[48]

Current statistics show ADE's from prescription drugs to be the number 4 killer in the United States of America. This will no doubt increase as false DTC advertising grows. Recognizing these inadequacies ensures that we do not fall victim to them.

ADE - Adverse drug Effects

---

[46] *The Lancet.* October 6, 2001;358:1141-1146.
      Graedon, Joe. Writing for L.A Daily Times. November 21, 2002.

[47] Kaisernetwork.org. *Health Policy as it Happens.* "Featured Issue: Direct-to-Consumer Prescription Drug Advertising."

[48] Testimony before the Subcommittee on Consumer Affairs Hearing, Senate Commerce Committee on Direct-to-Consumer (DTC) Advertising. (HRG Pubication #1583). Testimony of Sidney M. Wolfe, MD Director, Public Citizen's Health Research Group Senate Commerce Committee Subcommittee on Consumer Affairs Hearing on Direct-to-Consumer (DTC) Advertising. July 24, 2001.

Myth #3 – Pharmaceutical Drugs Improve the Quality of Human Life

Fact: When used as prescribed, prescription drugs kill more people than terrorism, car crashes, AIDS and street drugs combined.

Despite their overt social acceptance, pharmaceutical drugs are an expensive way to die. Thanks to Direct-to-Consumer Advertising (DTC Advertising), prescription drugs are often considered a Godsend. This belief has sparked a prescription drug "feeding frenzy." This can be seen by the measures that are taken by millions to ensure that they have continued access to these drugs, which can be rightfully considered poisons.

Millions of Americans pay for medical insurance each and every month of their lives simply to guarantee that they can snatch up a drug at any given point in time. Our senior citizens, who are far more susceptible to the dangers of prescription drugs, are secretly crossing the borders into Mexico or Canada to purchase their prescription drugs at discounted prices. To better accommodate this frenzy and their pharmaceutical money donors, the US Government strives to make

2001 - 140,6 billion on drugs

Shane Ellison M.Sc.

prescription drugs even more accessible via Medicare. Popularity of these drugs is surging every year. As reported by the *Kaiser Family Foundation, US spending for prescription drugs tripled between 1990 and 2001 to $140.6 billion and is expected to reach $445.9 billion dollars by 2012.*[49] To say that Americans are crazed for drugs is an understatement.

Paradoxically, this prescription drug "feeding frenzy" has caused worsening health amongst Americans. Authored by Barbara Starfield, MD, MPH, The *Journal of the American Medical Association (JAMA)* reported that by comparing 16 "health markers" considered indicative of good health, the United States ranks 12th out of the top 13 countries in regard to the health of its citizens.[50] These countries, listed in order of their ranking (with the first being the best) are Japan, Sweden, Canada, France, Australia, Spain, Finland, the Netherlands, the United Kingdom, the United States and Germany. In regards to the separate health indicators, the United States ranks as follows:

- 13th (last) for low birth weight percentages

- 13th for neonatal mortality and infant mortality overall

- 11th for post neonatal mortality

- 13th for years of potential life lost

- 11th for life expectancy at 1 year for females, 12th for males

US 13th in good health

Cohen, Jay, M.D. *Prescription Drug Use in America: The Startling Numbers And Their Implications.* http://www.medalternatives.com/articles/prescript_drug_use.html.

[50] *Journal of the American Chemical Society*, July 26, 2000-Vol 284, No.4.

40

- 10th for life expectancy at 15 years for females, 10th for males

- 10th for life expectancy at 40 years for females, 9th for males

- 7th for life expectancy at 65 years for females, 7th for males

- 3rd for life expectancy at 80 years for females, 3rd for males

- 10th for age-adjusted mortality

Most Americans have one foot in the grave. The Centers for Disease Control (CDC) reports that chronic diseases account for 7 out of every 10 deaths in the USA. Chronic diseases also account for more than 75% of medical care expenditures within the Unites States. Currently, at least 80% of seniors have at least one chronic disease and 50% have at least two.

In an attempt to avoid deteriorating health, or rather, in an attempt to remedy it, *American medical doctors write an average of 10 prescriptions per person every year.* Americans, like cattle, are lining up at the pharmaceutical trough for their dose of "just what the doctor ordered." Sadly, this addiction to prescription drugs has not led to better health. Instead, it has ignited an ungodly number of adverse drug reactions (ADRs), as documented by numerous peer-reviewed medical journals.

An ADR is defined as "any noxious, unintended and undesired effect of a drug, which occurs at doses used in humans for prophylaxis, diagnosis, or therapy."[51] Simply stated, an

---

[51] Lazarou, Jason, et al. "Incidence of Adverse Drug Reactions in Hospitalized Patients." *Journal of the American Medical Association.* April 15, 1998. Vol. 279, No. 15.

Shane Ellison M.Sc.

ADR is a negative side effect that occurs from using a drug as prescribed by a physician. Incidents involving errors in drug administration, noncompliance, drug abuse, overdose or therapeutic failure are not included in ADRs. Exclusion of these factors ensures that the number of ADRs from FDA approved drugs is not overestimated. Moreover, this conservative definition helps us to fully grasp the magnitude of ADRs associated with FDA approved drug use and the impact of ADRs on our health.

When studying the number of ADRs it is important to note the extreme difficulty in obtaining accurate figures. Many times, an ADR is not reported, is ignored, or is shrugged off as worsening health. It is estimated that only 15% of incidents that could have led to death or disability are reported by medical doctors, leaving 85% of ADR's to be silenced.[52] Hence, many experts feel that the following estimate for ADRs is conservative. To add to the difficulty, most studies of ADRs have been done in a hospital setting, thereby leaving out the number of ADRs that occur while patients sit at home watching football.

The study of ADRs began in the 1960s. During this time, it was estimated that 30% of those hospitalized suffered from ADRs and that 3% of hospitalizations were due to ADRs. Worse yet, in the 1960s it was estimated that there were 29,000 deaths annually due to ADRs.[53] By this estimate, 80 people died every day from taking FDA approved drugs exactly as they were prescribed. This is phenomenal in that this estimate from 1960 exceeds the number of people who currently die every year from illicit drug use! While a War on

[52] http://news.bbc.co.uk/go/pr/fr/-/1/hi/health/3840257.stm. Published: 2004/06/27 05:59:04 GMT © BBC MMIV.
[53] Classen, David. "Medication Safety. Moving from Illusion to Reality." *Journal of the American Medical Association*. March 5, 2003-Vol 289, No. 9.

Drugs (illicit drugs) has been declared, this problem, recognized over 40 years ago, was simply ignored.

The number of ADRs that occur today is staggering. The *New England Journal of Medicine* showed that ADRs occur in one out of every four individuals who visit their family medical doctor.[54] USA Today reported that the fourth leading cause of hospital admissions is from ADRs. It is estimated that 2.2 million Americans are so severely injured from FDA approved drugs that they are either hospitalized for long periods of time or permanently disabled.

Children are not immune to ADRs. Researchers writing for Pediatrics showed that between 1997 and 2000 there were 7,111 ADR reports on infants and children younger than age 2. Drug use was associated with an average of 243 reported deaths annually over the 38-month study period, with 100 (41%) occurring during the first month of life and 204 (84%) during the first year. In 1,432 (24%) of reported adverse event cases including all levels of severity, exposure to the drug was compliments of the mother during pregnancy, delivery, or lactation.[55] The FDA has stated that these numbers really only account for around 2% of the actual number of deaths and negative side effects reported!

This study, conducted by researchers at George Washington University, emphasizes the need for parents to think twice about administering drugs (and vaccines) to themselves while pregnant and to their infants. Parents must carefully weigh the risks versus benefits of medication and become more aware of natural alternatives for their children's health.

---

[54] Tejal K. Gandhi. et al. *Adverse Drug Events in Ambulatory Care.* Volume 348:1556-1564. April 17, 2003. Number 16.

[55] Moore TJ, Weiss SR, Kaplan S, Blaisdell CJ. "Reported adverse drug events in infants and children under 2 years of age." *Pediatrics.* 2002 Nov;110(5):e53.

not tested on children

The FDA does not require pharmaceutical companies to test newly released drugs for potentially hazardous effects on children. As a result, many, if not all, drugs are given to children without knowing whether or not they are safe. Still, prescription drug use by children is increasing more than any other age group. According to a study done in 2004, Yahoo News reports that we are drugging our youth twice as much, as can be seen by a 183% increase on spending for behavioral modifications for teenagers and by 369% in children aged 4 years or younger. FDA approved drugs are proving more dangerous than elicit drugs; forget about marijuana and alcohol, D.A.R.E. to keep your kids off of prescription drugs.

Side effects and injuries to other bodily systems from FDA approved drugs often require the consumer to take other prescription drugs in order to control the symptoms of the damage caused by the initial drug. In many cases, this means a lifetime of servitude to FDA approved drugs. Such servitude can severely limit a person's functional capabilities and decrease their lifespan.

The list of examples is nearly as long as the PDR; however, the following examples are the most glaring, occurring with great frequency in these commonly prescribed drugs.

Zyprexa (Olanzapine) is prescribed as an antidepressant and antipsychotic. The major side effect associated with using this drug (and other antidepressants and antipsychotics) is weight gain. Weight gain among users of Zyprexa is attributed to the fact that it slows the metabolism by blocking noradrenergic, dopamine, serotonin, and histamine receptors, all of which negatively affect metabolism and appetite control.[56]

---

[56] Wirshing A. Donna. et al. "Update on atypicals: Practical tips to manage common side effects." *Current Psychiatry Online*. Vol. 2, No. 3 / March 2003.

The subsequent weight gain from using Zyprexa results in an increased risk of hypertension, Type-II diabetes, coronary heart disease, stroke, gallbladder disease, osteoarthritis, and some forms of cancer. To ward off these side effects, the patient is often forced to take medications that are purported to decrease weight gain. Most notably, these include Wellbutrin and Meridia.

At best, Wellbutrin and Meridia lower body weight by 5%. As a result, there is no change in Body Mass Index (BMI). Therefore, many users will continue to suffer from the aforementioned risks associated with being overweight due to Zyprexa use *and* suffer from the negative side effects associated with Wellbutrin and Meridia. This inevitably forces users into a cycle of drug use, as medical doctors will be forced to prescribe secondary medication based on the side effects elicited by the weight gain from the initial drug, Zyprexa. This may be a lifetime of insulin use to control diabetes, blood thinners to prevent stroke, or NSAIDS to treat osteoarthritis (from excess weight). The list can be extensive and even culminate into the use of chemotherapy to ward off cancer, as the American Cancer Society (ACS) has stated that obesity may soon be the leading cause of cancer.

Prempro, which is made from the urine of pregnant mares just like its sister drug, Premarin, is a drug often prescribed for Hormone Replacement Therapy (HRT) for women who are post-menopausal or who have had a hysterectomy. On July 9, 2002, the National Institutes of Health (NIH) abruptly halted the use of Wyeth's Prempro in the Women's Health Initiative (WHI) because of the unacceptable risks associated with taking the drug. Sixteen thousand women received a letter advising them to stop taking Prempro.

The NIH letter explained that taking Prempro increases a woman's risk of breast cancer, heart disease, and stroke.[57] According to the National Heart, Lung and Blood Institute (NHLBI), women who were given Prempro were more likely to develop serious problems compared to those in the placebo group.

- 26% increase in breast cancer

- 41% increase in strokes

- 100% increase in blood clots

- 22% increase in incidents of cardiovascular disease

Further, Denise Grady, writing for The New York Times, reported that Hormone therapy doubled the risk of Alzheimer's disease and other types of dementia in women who began the treatment at age 65 or older.

Many patients who fell victim to HRT were forced into prescription drug servitude to simply maintain some semblance of health. To battle breast cancer, many medical doctors prescribe drugs such as Adriamycin (doxorubicin), Aredia (pamidronate disodium), Arimidex (anastrozole), Aromasin (exemestane), Chemotherapy Regimens, Cytoxan (cyclophosphamide), Ellence (epirubicin), Fareston (toremifene), Femara (letrozole), Herceptin (trastuzumab), Megace (megestrol), Tamoxifen, (Nolvadex), Taxol (paclitaxel), Taxotere (docetaxel), Xeloda (capecitabine), and Zoladex (goserelin acetate).[58] Of course, an array of other drugs is standing by to prevent

---

[57] *Patient Files First Nationwide Prempro Class Action Lawsuit Against Wyeth And Wyeth-Ayerst Research According to Schiffrin & Barroway, LLP; Wyeth Notifies Doctors and Pharmacists About Risks and Benefits Associated With Prempro.* July 16, 2002 12:36pm. BALA CYNWYD, Pa., July 16 /PRNewswire.

[58] http://imaginis.com/breasthealth/bc_drugs.asp.

stroke, blood clots and cardiovascular disease among users of HRT.

MMR - arthritis

The next example is particularly poignant as it affects our children. The MMR vaccine is a three-part vaccine, postulated to protect (immunize) against Measles, Mumps and German Measles (Rubella). As reported by *Clinical and Experimental Rheumatolology*, 55% of women who receive the Rubella/measles vaccine will suffer from rheumatoid arthritis.[59] This side effect from the MMR vaccine, which contains live viruses, is not surprising. Randall King, MD, of the Department of Emergency Medicine at the Medical College of Ohio has reported that one cause of rheumatoid arthritis is viral strains.[60]

Researchers writing for *Clinical and Experimental Rheumatolology* found that the rubella vaccine is associated with a number of arthritic reactions and recommended specifically that "those patients who have had an adverse reaction to rubella vaccination should be informed that they may seek compensation under the no-fault Vaccine Compensation Act, which is administered by the US Claims Court."

This real and present danger has not stopped the administration of this triple vaccine to both children and adults today. Many among the 55% of people who receive the vaccine and subsequently become victim to rheumatoid arthritis are destined to a lifetime of anti-rheumatic prescription drugs in an effort to become functional.

Ironically, those who are forced into a lifetime of drug use from previously using FDA approved drugs praise them

---

[59] Geier DA, Geier MR. "Rubella vaccine and arthritic adverse reactions: an analysis of the Vaccine Adverse Events Reporting System (VAERS) database from 1991 through 1998." *Clinical and Experimental Rheumatology*. 2001 Nov-Dec;19(6):724-6.

[60] http://www.emedicine.com/emerg/topic48.htm.

No fault Vaccine Compensation Act

adverse Drug Reactions (handwritten)

for their ability to maintain some semblance of functionality. While this is understandable, it is not logical, as they forget the primary reason for becoming a slave to prescription drugs. Further, their praise of FDA approved drugs inevitably elicits others to seek them out in order to fulfill hopes of achieving good health. Accordingly, they will suffer the same fate.

Worse than causing a lifetime of drug servitude, in addition to hospitalizing 2.2 million people every year, ADRs can also lead to death. In an attempt to calculate the number of deaths caused by ADRs, we look to the most authoritative medical journal in the world, the *Journal of the American Medical Association*. Entitled "Incidence of Adverse Drug Reactions in Hospitalized Patients", this study was a meta-analysis[61] of several studies over the last 32 years. This in-depth study concluded that there are an estimated 76,000-106,000 hospital deaths each year directly caused by ADRs. This is a far cry from the 1960s! This statistic alone ranks ADRs somewhere between the fourth and sixth leading cause of death in America, yet does not account for the number of deaths outside of the hospital.[62]

To bring this death toll into perspective, 106,000 deaths per year equates to one individual dying every five minutes from "approved" drugs. This averages out to 300 people dying every day...twice as many deaths in a single year as the total number of deaths from the Vietnam War. Moreover, these

---

[61] A meta-analysis is a statistical procedure to combine a number of existing studies. Through such a procedure, effects that are hard or impossible to discern in the original studies because of a too-small sample size can be made visible, as the meta-analysis is (in the ideal case) equivalent to a single study with the combined size of all original studies. A weakness of the method is that problems with any of the studies will affect the result of the meta-analysis, so a good meta-analysis of bad studies will still result in bad data.

[62] *Journal of the American Chemical Society*, July 26, 2000-Vol 284, No.4.

300 people die a day from approved drugs (handwritten)

deaths far outnumber those caused by car accidents, AIDS, alcohol, illicit drug use, infectious diseases, diabetes, and murder combined.[63, 64] If this trend continues over the next ten years, FDA approved drugs will kill an estimated one million people.

To reiterate, these statistics DO NOT include deaths caused by administrative or medical error (medication error, drug abuse and deaths caused by taking more or less of a drug than the prescribed amount) or those outside of the hospital! Today, many experts are using the term adverse drug event (ADE) to describe the negative side effects and deaths from medication errors. Thus, in contrast to ADRs, the definition of ADEs includes errors in administration.

ADE

The distinction between ADRs and ADEs is an important one. Most, if not all health professionals are attributing the 106,000 deaths caused by drugs to administrative error. This seriously discounts the dangers of prescription drugs due to the fact that those who don't make the distinction will ignore the dangers of FDA approved drugs and simply attempt to find better ways of prescribing drugs. While this may lower the number of errors, it will not affect the 100,000 deaths that occur every year from FDA approved drugs in the form of ADRs. Most likely, this lazy thinking will only contribute to the FDA approved drug holocaust (if 100,000 people dying every year is not a holocaust, what is?).

Looking at ADEs from FDA approved drugs gives a much larger picture of the consequences of "following doctor's orders." In 1999, the Institute of Medicine estimated that 98,000 people a year die from adverse drug events. This rate

---

[63] Lazarou, Jason. Pomeranz, H. Bruce. Corey, Paul. " Incidence of Adverse Drug Reactions in Hospitalized Patients." *Journal of the American Medical Association*, April 15, 1998. Vol. 279, No. 15.

[64] Cohen, S. Jay. *Over Dose*. 2001. ISBN 1-58542-123-5.

appears to have grown. Extrapolating from an editorial published in *JAMA* on March 5th of 2003 by David Classen, MD, MS, we find that as many as 1,900,000 ADE's occur annually among the Medicare population! As many as 180,000 of these ADE's are life threatening or fatal! In his closing, Dr. Classen notes that this estimate is conservative.[65] Still growing, Reuters showed that in 2004, Colorado-based HealthGrades Inc. surveyed hospitals in all 50 states and discovered that ADEs contributed to a jaw-dropping 195,000 deaths in US hospitals.[66]

Nevertheless, parents rush their children to the hospital at the smallest sign of illness, millions of the elderly are scrambling for drugs, and men are begging for cholesterol lowering drugs because "Joe" at work saw a commercial about how effective they are while watching football and drinking beer. Whether they are jumping the border or begging their congressman for drug discounts, Americans erroneously believe that prescription drugs will help them. Once again, this exposes the true power of DTC advertising.

While the FDA may set laws governing the use of medicine and nutritional supplements, they are far from setting the standards of what is right and wrong.

That companies are profiting from drugs that kill hundreds of thousands is, in its most precise definition, a crime against humanity. People have been imprisoned and killed for less.

Those who are directly affected by FDA approved drugs do seek justice. Many victims or those family members of the deceased, attempt to seek justice in the courts by suing manu-

[65] Moride Y, et al. *British Journal of Clinical Pharmacology*. 1997; 43:177-181.
[66] Reuters. *Report Says 195,000 Deaths Due to Hospital Error*. http://reuters.com/newsArticle.jhtml?type=healthNews&storyID=5790535.

facturers such as Eli Lilly and Pfizer. But thanks to the Bush administration, this is not an option.

The Bush administration has been going to court to halt lawsuits by consumers who say they have been injured by FDA approved drugs. Downplaying the devastation of FDA approved drugs and shielding drug manufacturers from damage suits, the Bush administration asserts that allowing consumers to sue manufacturers would "undermine public health" and interfere with federal regulation of drugs.[67]

In sharp contrast to this, purveyors of nutritional supplements are raided and imprisoned for simply making so called "false health claims" for their products. In line with this bias, nutritional supplements are labeled dangerous and ineffective. Though, in a letter to Senator Hillary Clinton, Consumers Health Freedom Coalition shows that in 2002, The American Association of Poison Control Centers' (AAPCC) annual report documented a mere 11 deaths total from the improper use of nutritional supplements. Important to clarify, these 11 deaths were from people using nutritional supplements outside of their recommended use, and most striking in 2002, the AAPCC only recorded 1 death from the wrongful use of the herb ephedra. In appalling contrast to this, and remember that FDA approved drugs caused over 100,000 deaths every year, not from errors but from properly used drugs taken as directed. This trend is estimated to have continued over the last 30 years.

Ignoring the body count, medical doctors are so hypnotized by drug propaganda that they demand more drugs. Despite the documented dangers of prescription drugs, if drug approval slows and there is a subsequent lack of newly ap-

---

[67]   Pear, Robert. "In a Shift, Bush Moves to Block Medical Suits." *The New York Times. July 25, 2004.*

proved drugs available, the *Student British Medical Journal* reports that medical doctors consider it a "crisis."[68] Answering to this false crisis, in addition to shielding drug manufacturers from damage suits, the Unites States government has strived to decrease drug approval times in an effort to get them to market quicker! The United States Department of Health and Human services Secretary Tommy G. Thompson emphatically states that the "FDA is making new treatments available more quickly, and I expect FDA's new innovation initiatives announced early in 2003 will lead to even faster approvals of safe and affordable medical treatments in the coming years."

21ˢᵗ Century Medicine

Drug company designs new drug. Drug company funds and designs clinical trials. Drug company interprets and relays results to medical doctors. Medical doctors become engorged with excitement. Drug gains FDA approval. Drug company spends more money on advertising the new drug than on researching it. Drug is prescribed by medical doctors. Medical doctors and drug company get paid.

Patient dies. Evidence shows that drug killed patient. US Government does not allow patient's family to sue. Death certificate of deceased patient reads heart attack. Patient's family goes on antidepressants. Medical doctors and pharmaceutical companies make more money. US Government works tirelessly to approve more drugs at an even faster rate for their pharmaceutical clients. Purveyors of nutritional supplements are jailed.

In support of this idiocy, the most common argument in favor of using FDA approved drugs is that, when looking at

---

[68] http://www.studentbmj.com/back_issues/0203/news/8.html.

work only in 30 65 70

the "big picture," the benefits derived from or the effectiveness of FDA approved drugs justify the risk. This is an ill thought-out hypothesis. Outside of "emergency medicine," rarely, if at all, is this true. While prescription drugs are estimated to be the number four killer in the United States of America, the majority of them are absolutely ineffective in that they offer no benefit whatsoever.[69] Despite the multi-billion dollar ad campaigns, the media coverage, and the deceptively-written articles found in the medical journals which praise the benefits of prescription drugs; the vast majority of drugs only work for 30-50% of the population, as confessed by Glaxo Chief Allen Roses. Therefore, in many cases, there is all risk, and no benefit. This is hardly a good argument in favor of FDA approved drug use!

For every loser there is always a winner. Massive profit from negative side effects is the primary reason, whether openly admitted to or not, that very little is being done to curb the death toll from FDA approved drugs. In addition to profiting on the upfront sales of FDA approved drugs, pharmaceutical companies and their client, the FDA (via the Prescription Drug User Fee Act), are also making billions from the negative side effects they elicit amongst users.

To obtain an accurate measurement of just how much negative side effects caused by FDA approved drugs really costs Americans, a mathematical model was developed and published in *Archives of Internal Medicine*. This study showed that drug-related morbidity and mortality is costing Americans an astonishing $76 billion per year![70]

---

[69] Connor, Steve. "Glaxo chief: Our drugs do not work on most patients." *Independent.co.uk.* 12/8/03.

[70] Johnson JA, Bootman JL. "Drug-related morbidity and mortality. A cost-of-illness model." *Archives of Internal Medicine.* 1995;155:1949-1956.

Shane Ellison M.Sc.

benefits from side effects

The beneficiaries of these $76 billion dollars are the already wealthy pharmaceutical companies and doctors. It works like this: Your doc (yes, the family doc who everybody loves) unknowingly prescribes a dangerous drug and you suffer more from the drug than you did from the sickness. Consequently, rather than attribute your new symptoms to negative side effects, you are diagnosed with a new illness. As a result, you begin taking other drugs or are hospitalized in an unsuccessful attempt to ward off the new illness (remember, in reality you are being treated for the negative side effects associated with the initial prescription drug). All the while, your doc and the pharmaceutical companies extrapolate an extra $300 every year from those who have become ill from FDA approved drugs. This equates to an extra $76 billion dollars in profit.

This money also spreads to the stock market. As reported in Public Citizen, while profits of Fortune 500 companies declined by 53% [in 2001], the top US drug makers had an increase in profits of 33%![71] Whether it is your friendly family doctor or the next-door neighbor who is financing his second home with pharmaceutical stock options, millions of people are making money from FDA approved drugs. These same millions of people are looking away in an effort to ignore the facts and maximize their gains. What good is being rich if you are dead?

With respect to those who profit from the pain of others, such as the FDA and the pharmaceutical companies, Jay R. Cavanaugh, PhD, Member, California State Board of Pharmacy 1980-90 states:

"This collection of serial killers with reckless disregard of human life, extinguishes the hopes and lives of over 100,000 Americans every year. In the past decade they

---

[71] *Public Citizen.* April 18th, 2002.

have been responsible for over one million innocent deaths, yet not only have they not faced justice, they have enriched themselves with profits that would make Bill Gates envious. These parasitic killers come not from some cave in Afghanistan, but from plush office suites..."[72]

The grip of the pharmaceutical industry on drug research helps to explain why deadly drugs are approved in the first place. When it comes to drug research (*in vitro*, animal or human clinical trials), drug companies often design the protocol, choose the investigators and in many instances, are involved in the collation, interpretation and reporting of data. According to *The Lancet*, rarely are negative results from drug research reported. Instead, drug companies are publishing only the positive results from their studies in an attempt to increase popularity and get their drugs to market.[73] Recognizing this conflict of interest, *The Lancet* accused pharmaceutical companies of "confusion, manipulation and institutional failure."[74] Such deceit is the tip of the iceberg, and as we will see in chapter 4; the pharmaceutical industry goes to even greater lengths to push their drugs.

Before you "follow doctor's orders," use this simple test to see if the prescription is right for you or your children, it may save your life by preventing ADE's and ADR's!

- Do not look at promotional brochures, which often contain unpublished material, misleading graphs, and selective quotations.

---

[72] Cavanaugh Jay R. Editorial entitled "Reckless Disregard." Posted at DrugWar.com January 21, 2003.

[73] Collier, Joe. Iheanacho, Ike. "The Pharmaceutical Industry as an Informant." *Lancet* 2002; 360: 1405-09.

[74] *BBC News*. "Negative drug research 'withheld.'" Friday, 23 April, 2004.

- Ignore anecdotal evidence, such as the fact that celebrities recommend the product.

- Use the **NEST** acronym when questioning your doctor.

  - **Natural Alternatives** – Are there any natural alternatives that you are aware of? Most drugs are derived from natural products. Hence, in many cases you can find a safe and inexpensive alternative. If your doctor cannot help you, consider visiting a health food store or naturopathic doctor before filling the prescription.

  - **Efficacy** – How many studies have shown the drug to be effective?

  - **Safety** – What is the likelihood of long-term or serious side effects caused by the drug? (Remember that safety of new drugs is poorly documented)

  - **Tolerability** – What are the withdraw rates of the drug? In other words, how many people quit taking the drug during clinical trials? Your doctor, through the company sales representative, can easily discover this. If the drop out rate is high… beware, it is not tolerable!

Myth #4 – Professional Medicine Reporting is Honest and Trustworthy

Fact: The pharmaceutical industry's influence over the medical profession is the basis for false reporting of drug safety and benefits.

The power and sophistication of the pharmaceutical industry's grip on professional medicine reporting sets the tone among professionals surrounding FDA approved drugs. Various tactics of persuasion are used in an attempt to increase popularity of a drug among medical doctors, despite a lack of safety and effectiveness. This persuasion by the pharmaceutical industry has a dark history of outright lies, deception and half-truths that ultimately put the patient at great risk.

Medical doctors rely on "peer-reviewed medical journals" to learn about the advances in modern medicine. Most notably, these journals include the *Lancet, British Medical Journal (BMJ), New England Journal of Medicine (NEJM)* and the *Journal of the American Medical Association (JAMA)*. It is thought that due to the rigorous scientific standards required for publication, that these journals offer the hard science behind any given drug. Thus, having a trained eye, medical doctors feel confident that they are able to decide whether any given drug is safe and effective for their clients after reading these journals.

Unfortunately, utilizing medical journals to decipher whether a drug is safe and effective is becoming virtually impossible. This is due to drug company sponsored "ghost writing" and "checkbook science." While you may have never heard of these terms, you will definitely want to know about them, as they have insurmountable affects on your health. Ghost writing and checkbook science are how medical doctors are falsely convinced that FDA approved drugs are safe and effective.

With billions of dollars at their disposal, pharmaceutical companies engage in a little-known secret referred to as "Medical Ghost Writing." Medical ghost writing can rightly be considered "one of the biggest medical deceptions in history." As reported by Erica Johnson of CBC news, medical ghostwriting is the practice of hiring PhDs to crank out favorable drug reports, purposefully leaving out negative side effects, for drug companies. Once the report is complete, drug companies recruit doctors to put their name on the report as the authors. These reports are then published in the most prestigious medical journals, such as the *Lancet, British Medical Journal,* and *New England Journal of Medicine.*[75] The carrot for this deceitful practice is money. For their efforts, ghostwriters can receive up to $20,000 per report, while medical doctors are enticed with both money and prestige. Needless to say, this is an unimaginable "conflict of interest."

As deplorable as medical ghost writing sounds, it is more common than you think. Let us look to the world's most in-

---

[75] Johnson, Erica. "Medical Ghostwriting." *CBC News.* Mar 25, 2003.

fluential medical journal, the *New England Journal of Medicine*, as an example. The *NEJM* has admitted that ghostwriters, who received an undisclosed amount of financial support from the pharmaceutical companies to formulate the reviews, have written 50% of drug therapy reviews published in their journal. Dr. Jeffrey Drazen, the *New England Journal's* editor, insists that pharmaceutical money reaches so far that he simply can't find experts to write for him that do not have financial ties to the drugs they were writing about.

Thus, the drug companies' financial force in peer reviewed medical journals allows them to dominate popular thinking among both practicing medical doctors and academic physicians when it comes to drug safety and effectiveness. As a result, many doctors unknowingly prescribe ineffective, overtly expensive or life threatening drugs. Ultimately, thanks to medical ghost writing:

- You get biased advice regarding prescription drugs. Often times, strengths of a drug are highlighted while weaknesses are left out.

- The treatment you get is skewed by drug company influence.

- Many times, the prescription you get is several times more expensive than other equally effective drugs.

- And sometimes, your prescription is not even the right drug at all.

To better illustrate the negative impact of medical ghostwriting, we look to Dr. M. Michael Wolfe. As a medical expert, the editors of the *Journal of the American Medical Association* (*JAMA*) sent him an unpublished drug review on the arthritis medication Celebrex to evaluate. At first glance, he was impressed by what he read. It appeared that after six months

Shane Ellison M.Sc.

of a company-sponsored study involving more than 8,000 patients, the drug was associated with lower rates of stomach and intestinal ulcers than two older arthritis medicines, diclofenac and ibuprofen. Feeling confident that the drug was safe, Dr. Wolfe and colleagues wrote a favorable editorial about Celebrex to accompany the newly released findings in *JAMA*. Consequently, millions of MDs began prescribing the now commonly used Celebrex.

As time passed, it was learned, that like many medical doctors of today, Dr. Wolf was a victim of ghostwriting. As fate would have it, Dr. Wolfe eventually came across the complete data from the same study as a member of the FDA's arthritis advisory committee. He saw numerous discrepancies between the initial report and the newly found raw data. Most notably, Pharmacia, the manufacturers of Celebrex, made it appear as if the study lasted only 6 months. In reality, the study of Celebrex lasted a year. During the last half of the year (which was unreported) almost all of the ulcer complications that occurred during the study were in Celebrex users. When all of the data was considered, Dr. Wolfe stated that most of Celebrex's apparent safety advantages disappeared.

Unfortunately, *JAMA* had already released the previously written findings that were derived from the fabricated report, along with Dr. Wolf's favorable editorial. In an effort to discover why the initial report did not illustrate the entire findings of the study, Dr. Wolfe found that the study's 16 authors included faculty members of eight medical schools. All authors were either employees of Pharmacia or paid consultants of the company.[76]

The ghostwritten lies behind NSAIDS and disregard for patients' health worsens. Between 1990 and 1997, all clini-

---

[76] Okie, Susan. *Washington Post*, August 5, 2001; Page A11.

cal trials performed on non-steroidal anti-inflammatory drugs (NSAIDS) such as Aleve, aspirin, Motrin, Ibuprofen, valdecoxib – Bextra®, celecoxib – Celebrex®, diclofenac – Voltaren®, etodolac – Lodine®, fenoprofen – Nalfon®, indomethacin – Indocin®, ketoprofen – Orudis®, Oruvail®, ketoralac – Toradol®, oxaprozin – Daypro®, nabumetone – Relafen®, sulindac – Clinoril®, tolmetin – Tolectin®, and rofecoxib – Vioxx® were sponsored by the drug manufacturers. The result was that 100% of the studies showed the sponsored drug to have equal or superior efficacy when compared to other drugs.[77] Thus, according to studies done from 1990-1997, every NSAID drug tested during this time was superior to every other NSAID product...all at the same time.

The fallacies behind medical ghost writing on NSAIDS are quickly exposed through an increasing number of deaths among users. Despite the fabricated studies showing NSAIDS to be safe, real-life observations show that approximately 107,000 patients are hospitalized every year for non-steroidal anti-inflammatory drug-related gastrointestinal complications. Moreover, at least 16,500 NSAID-related deaths occur each year among arthritis patients.[78] This figure, as reported by Dr. Gurkirpal Singh, is comparable to the number of deaths from the acquired immunodeficiency syndrome [AIDS] and shows that NSAIDS contribute to as many deaths as multiple myeloma, asthma, and cervical cancer combined! Adding to the devastation, the risk of miscarriage for women who take aspirin is 60 percent higher than for those who do not.

Although outrageously high, the aforementioned statistics do not account for over-the-counter use of NSAIDS, only

[77] Ivan Oransky and Jeanne Lenzer. "Ties to drug manufacturers deform medical reviews." *USA Today*. McLean, Va.:Aug1, 2002. Page A11.
[78] Singh Gurkirpal, MD, "Recent Considerations in Nonsteroidal Anti-Inflammatory Drug Gastropathy", *The American Journal of Medicine*. July 27, 1998, p. 31S.

for arthritis patients. Thus, we can be confident that there are considerably more deaths caused by the use of NSAIDS that go unreported. And because few medical doctors are unaware of these statistics, NSAIDS can rightfully be considered a silent killer, especially when "experts" are paid to write favorable reviews and drug manufacturers carry out their own clinical studies. If NSAIDS were not a silent killer, you would see publicity seeking, Hollywood stars holding fundraisers for NSAIDS victims, not AIDS victims.

Being unaware of this silent killer, millions of Americans are consuming NSAIDS on a daily basis on the false hypothesis that they will successfully enhance their longevity. This will go down in the history books as one of America's deadliest medical errors. How many people do you know who take an aspirin a day in an attempt to lower their risk of heart disease? What about Celebrex? Vioxx?

Utilizing their billions of expendable dollars, many drug companies have published ghostwritten articles in peer-reviewed medical journals in an attempt to rave about their newest drug. These drug companies and their drugs include, but are not limited to, AstraZeneca and Omeprazol, Pfizer and Zoloft and Warner Lambert and Neurontin. We can be confident that many other companies are guilty as well. Posted on the *British Medical Journal* website, ex-medical ghostwriter Susanna Rees stated that:

> "Medical writing agencies go to great lengths to disguise the fact that the papers they ghostwrite and submit to journals and conferences are ghostwritten on behalf of pharmaceutical companies and not by the named authors,' she wrote. 'There is a relatively high success rate for ghostwritten submissions - not outstanding, but consistent."[79]

---

[79] Barnett, Antony. Public Affairs Editor. Sunday December 7, 2003. *The Observer.*

Other ghostwriters have come forward privately to offer testimony:

Ghostwriter 1

"I agreed to do two reviews for a supplement to appear under the names of respected 'authors.' I was given an outline, references, and a list of drug-company approved phrases. I was asked to sign an agreement stating that I would not disclose anything about the project. I was pressured to rework my drafts to position the product more favorably."

Ghostwriter 2

"I was told exactly what the drug company expected and given explicit instructions about what to play up and what to play down."

The editor of the *British Journal of Medicine* has acknowledged that medical ghostwriting has become a serious problem:

"'We are being hoodwinked by the drug companies. The articles come in with doctors' names on them and we often find some of them have little or no idea about what they have written."

"Scientists at the Hershey's Center for Obesity Research have concluded that eating a chocolate bar once daily actually reduces your chances of getting fat!" Well, this is obviously made up. However, this kind of company-backed research is becoming far too common among drug companies and is undermining the trust in science held by medical doctors.

While the art of mass deception through medical ghostwriting is promulgated to medical doctors, pharmaceutical companies also work vigorously to falsely perpetuate drug popularity by sponsoring its own drug research by paying university researchers. Going into the halls of academia to crush science as we know it and rebuild anew, drug companies will conveniently sponsor their own drug research by paying university researchers in order to gain drug popularity. This is commonly referred to as "checkbook science." As defined by Diana Zuckerman PhD, checkbook science is research intended not to expand knowledge or to benefit humanity, but instead to sell products [drugs]. Checkbook science has stolen the very soul of University research, scientific method, and the patients who serve as human subjects. [80]

Like medical ghostwriting, checkbook science is far more common than you think. Shannon Brownlee, writing for Washington Monthly, has stated, "for the past two decades, medical research has been quietly corrupted by cash from private [Drug] industry."

While it may be kept quiet, a few astute researchers have noticed the negative impact of checkbook science. According to research performed by Bekelman and associates, the halls of academia are being flooded with pharmaceutical money in an attempt to control the outcome of pharmaceutical research. Their study, published in the prestigious *Journal of the American Medical Association,* found that about a third of investigators at academic institutions had personal financial ties with industry sponsors. Furthermore, in addition to direct payments, these researchers show the relatively new phenomenon of academic institutions holding equity in pharmaceutical companies for future payout once the drug company "hits it big" with their new drug!

---

[80] Zuckerman D. "Hype in health reporting: "checkbook science" buys distortion of medical news." *International Journal of Health Services.* 2003;33(2).

Many argue that checkbook science does not affect the outcome of drug research. Fortunately, Bekelman and associates refute this argument in their published research. When assessing the impact of checkbook science, the authors found that a review of 1,140 articles showed that industry sponsored studies "were significantly more likely to show favorable conclusions relative to non-industry studies."[81]

Favorable conclusions among drug industry sponsored studies were attributed to two factors. First, industry-sponsored study designs had a higher tendency to give positive results by using a placebo rather than using comparison therapies in controlled trials. Secondly, industry-sponsored studies routinely failed to publish negative data found by researchers. In laymen's terms, drug companies were able to design the study in such a way that it would show favorable results. Second, if this failed to show favorable results then the negative data was simply discarded! Checkbook science at its best!

Checkbook science has been considered the greatest danger to public health. Heart drugs serve as an excellent example. Heart drugs prescribed for abnormal heart rhythm were introduced in the late seventies. By 1990, they were estimated to kill more Americans than the Vietnam War. Early research suggested these drugs were lethal, which would have saved thousands of lives. Yet, these research findings went unpublished by the pharmaceutical company who paid for the research.[82]

Most recently, researchers for the National Institute for Clinical Excellence (NICE) strived to develop guidelines for

[81] Bekelman, J.E., Li, Y. and Gross, C. P. "Scope and impact of financial conflicts of interest in biomedical research." *Journal of the American Medical Association.* 289, 454-465.

[82] Jeremy Laurence. Health Editor. "Pharmaceutical companies accused of manipulating drug trials for profit." *Independent.co.uk.*

prescribing antidepressant drugs, known as Selective Serotonin Reuptake Inhibitors (SSRIs), to children. In their endeavors, they approached drug companies for their research findings. NICE researchers report that they were denied access to this vital information.

Published evidence by the pharmaceutical companies showed SSRIs to be safe and effective for children. Conversely though, when unpublished results were finally obtained from independent researchers, it was discovered that there was an increased risk of suicidal ideas and attempted suicide among users of antidepressants. Accurately reported, the *British Medical Journal* shows that children taking antidepressants are twice as likely to become suicidal as children taking placebo.[83]

Specifically, the SSRI drug known as Paxil (paroxetine) and its maker GlaxoSmithKline has come under attack for hiding unpublished studies surrounding the dangers of its use on children. Eliot Spitzer, Attorney General for New York State, has filed a lawsuit against GlaxoSmithKline, claiming that they suppressed studies that its leading antidepressant increases suicidal tendencies among children. Apparently, 2 million Paxil prescriptions were written to children in 2002 while GlaxoSmithKline kept trial results from the public and its sales force.

GlaxoSmithKline has denied any wrongdoing. Despite the company's defense, medical authorities in both the US and the UK have banned doctors from prescribing the drug to anyone less than 18 years of age. Considering that over 2 million prescriptions were written and that GlaxoSmithKline profited $250 million in sales of Paxil to children, it is a bit late.[84] Big

[83] Lenzer, Jeanne. Secret US report surfaces on antidepressants in children. BMJ 2004;329:307 (7 August)
[84] Foley, Stephen. "Glaxo Sued Over Paxil Child Suicides." *The Independent – UK.* June 03, 2004.

Pharma always wins. Most fitting is the statement published in the medial journal *The Lancet*: "The story of research into SSRI use in childhood depression is one of confusion, manipulation, and institutional failure."[85]

Checkbook science is not only common among Universities. It appears that the wallet of Big Pharma extends all the way to the top...National Institutes of Health. Called the "Stealth Merger" by *the LA Times*, we find that top scientists at the National Institutes of Health collect paychecks and stock options from the drug industry, in secret.[86] Once considered "an island of objective and pristine research, untainted by the influences of commercialization," the National Institutes of Health has become tainted by "checkbook science" as can be seen from the following statistics from *the LA Times*:

- Dr. Stephen I. Katz, director of the NIH's National Institute of Arthritis and Musculoskeletal and Skin Diseases collected between $476,369 and $616, 365 in fees over a ten-year period.

- From 1997-2002, Dr. John I. Gallin, director of the NIH's Clinical Center, received between $145,000 and $322,000 in fees and stock proceeds from the drug industry.

- Dr. Richard C. Eastman is the NIH's top diabetes researcher. As a consultant to the drug manufacturers in 1997, he wrote to the Food and Drug Administration defending a product without disclosing his conflict of interest. His letter stated that the risk of liver failure

---

[85] "DATA FROM UNPUBLISHED TRIALS SUGGEST THAT MOST SSRI ANTIDEPRESSANT DRUGS UNSUITABLE FOR CHILDREN" (pp 1335, 1341) *Lancet* 2004; 363: 1335, 1341-45.

[86] Willman, David. LA Times Staff Writer. "Stealth Merger: Drug Companies and Government Medical Research." December 7, 2003.

from the given drug was "very minimal." Six months later, a patient taking the drug in an NIH study that Eastman oversaw, Audrey LaRue Jones, suffered sudden liver failure and died. An autopsy, along with liver experts, found that the drug had caused the liver failure.

- Dr. Ronald N. Germain, deputy director of a major laboratory at the National Institute of Allergy and Infectious Diseases, amassed more than $1.4 million in company consulting fees from 1993 to 2003, plus stock options.

- Jeffrey Schlom, director of the National Cancer Institute's Laboratory of Tumor Immunology and Biology, received $331,500 in company fees over 10 years.

- Jeffrey M. Trent, who became scientific director of the National Human Genome Research Institute in 1993, reported between $50,608 and $163,000 in industry consulting fees. He left the government in 2002.

NIH officials now allow more than 95% of the agency's top-paid employees to keep these "consulting" fees confidential. In fact, the NIH is the most secretive agency in the US government when it comes to disclosing financial conflicts of interest.

Pharmaceutical companies with potential massive financial gains have clearly found a loophole by which they can manipulate research in a way such that they are able to produce positive research results and subsequently make a profit, and a humungous one at that. The flood of money from drug research guarantees that the truth behind synthetic drugs remains hidden from medical doctors. Checkbook science shows us why they often accept the myth that "FDA approved drugs are safe and effective." Meanwhile, millions of people suffer from the deadly side effects associated with prescription drugs.

How to Be a Corporate Drug Dealer

The growth in knowledge of biochemistry, physiology, organic chemistry, and chemical process methods has yielded millions of new synthetic (man-made) drug targets. These new discoveries have the potential to bring billion-dollar profits to any pharmaceutical company that can convince medical doctors, the FDA and the American public of the necessity of these new patentable drugs in ensuring health. Considering that these drugs have toxicity profiles that make marijuana and crack look like candy and that natural, inexpensive medicine derived from food is easily accessible and extremely effective, this endeavor looks impossible at first glance.

However, I want to make it clear to my fellow pharmaceutical entrepreneurs that several proven methods for success in corporate drug dealing exist. These methods are readily available to us, and have proven so effective that if done properly, naïve Americans will be begging us for the latest and greatest synthetic drug. More exciting, once used, their blind loyalty to our drugs will undoubtedly lead to further drug use as a means for treating the negative side effects associated with the initial drug we push on these fools. So, go by a new house, hell, buy two. Buy your wives a vacation to a tropical island. Get your teenage kids a new SUV. Pay cash for your new Lexus and private jet. While the stock market drops at record speeds, our profits will be soaring. In no time, we will have an amount of money that would make every industry in the world envious. Ready? Listen closely now:

First and foremost, we must gain the trust of medical doctors. They haven't been trained on the use of natural medicine for over 75 years, so convincing them of the importance that our drugs carry will be like feeding candy to a baby.

The second secret is known as "Medical Ghostwriting." In order to convince doctors that our drugs are extremely safe and effective we will find academic PhDs (poor, hungry and driven) to write favorable reports about our drugs. Considering that these reports will be false it is unlikely that the PhDs will be willing to put their names on the papers, and may even be reluctant to write them. To push them into doing what we say, we'll offer them $20,000 for each report! Don't worry; this is pennies compared to what we'll make. And considering how overworked and underpaid these PhDs are, they'll beg us for the opportunity.

Since they won't put their names on the false reports, we'll simply find complacent, high-paid doctors (a dime a dozen) looking for prestige to list their names as authors. Once done, we'll publish these reports in peer-reviewed medical journals like the *Lancet, British Medical Journal,* and *New England Journal of Medicine.* Other medical doctors will read these and succumb to the scientifically written propaganda and ultimately begin feeding our drugs to the public!

Third, we want the public to go along with the charade and eat whatever drug the medical doctors feed them. To this end, we will deceitfully and tirelessly advertise directly to all of America via radio, magazine and television. We'll secretly call this guerrilla drug marketing and do it under the guise of "promoting better health and drug awareness" and publicly call it Direct-to-Consumer Advertising. Every single ad will focus on how safe and effective our drugs are. We'll throw in a few antidotal negative side effects to make the ad appear "more real."

I assure you, this type of Direct-to-Consumer advertising is the Holy Grail for success in corporate drug pushing.

According to the United States General Accounting Office (GAO), drugs that are promoted directly to consumers are often the best-selling drugs, despite their lack of safety and effectiveness. As shown by the GAO in its report to congress, sales for DTC advertised drugs increase faster than sales for drugs that are not heavily advertised to consumers. Specifically, between 1999 and 2000, the number of prescription drugs dispensed that underwent heavy DTC advertising rose 25 percent. Conversely, drugs that did not undergo heavy DTC advertising only increased 4 percent. In no time, these gullible, hamburger-eating Americans will be thanking God for our drugs and will be depending on them, rather than diet and lifestyle habits, for health and longevity.

Over time, taking our drugs and becoming an FDA-approved drug addict will be the norm. In fact, becoming an FDA-approved drug addict will be so commonplace that refusal of our drugs will make one look like a "fool." We can then convince all of America that alternative health practitioners who promote natural medicine are "quacks" with no scientific basis whatsoever for their claims.

Future tactics can be employed if necessary, there's nothing wrong with being greedy. Once the aforementioned techniques are in place we can begin other routes of guerrilla drug pushing. For instance:

- We can invent diseases characterized by common everyday symptoms.

- We can convince parents that their kids should be docile robots and if not, then they must feed them central nervous system stimulants to make them "normal" (we will define normal).

- We can brainwash the public into thinking that everyone should have the exact same cholesterol levels or face the consequence of early death, thus causing them to take our cholesterol-lowering drugs. I know, this one sounds crazy but I guarantee we can make it work.

- We can even elicit the help of the DEA to make natural drugs illegal to possess. This will force the more intelligent persons to take our drugs as a last ditch effort to procure health rather than taking inexpensive natural medicine.

- And finally, we can engage armies of pharmaceutical reps onto the front lines by having them visit every single medical doctor in the nation to distribute our drug propaganda. These reps will be paid handsomely, as to curb any ethical or moral reservation they might have about dealing our drugs.

Who said getting rich wasn't easy? This is going to be a breeze, especially when you're dealing with an obese and complacent audience! Celebrate good times, C'mon! Oh, and whatever you do, DO NOT take these drugs for yourself!

Guaranteed Natural Joint Relief for Osteoarthritis

Typically, joint pain is caused by osteoarthritis, which is estimated to affect 50 million Americans mostly age 40 and up. Understanding joint pain affords us the ability to treat it properly.

Studies show that osteoarthritis is the result of our body lacking the ability to manufacture a molecule known as glucosamine (perhaps due to age, poor diet or genetics). This inability to manufacture glucosamine leads to a lack of collagen.

Collagen is the protein portion of the fibrous substance that holds joints together. It is also the main component of the shock-absorbing cushion called articular cartilage, the white, smooth surface that covers the ends of body joints. These cushions can be found in the wrist, fingers, toes, ankles, knees, hips and between the discs of the spine. Without articular cartilage, our joints experience pain and despite how healthy we may be, this pain greatly inhibits physical activity. Lack of physical activity inevitably leads to a decline in health.

The obvious first step towards treating this pain and to prevent the subsequent decline in health is to provide the body with an orally active form (one that can make it past the stomach and into the blood stream) of glucosamine. After decades of research, scientists have found this to be glucosamine sulfate rather than glucosamine HCL.

Glucosamine sulfate is derived from chitin, which is a processed form of shrimp, lobster, and crab shells. Glucosamine sulfate is a derivative of the naturally occurring aminomonosaccharide glucosamine, a major constituent of cartilage and synovial fluid. When supplemented properly (1500-2500 mg daily for 6-8 weeks) glucosamine sulfate rebuilds lost cartilage and soothes joints. In an unprecedented, 3-year, randomized, placebo-controlled, double blind study involving 200 patients, supplementation with glucosamine sulfate retarded the progression of osteoarthritis in the knee. Other studies have confirmed these findings by showing that supplementation with glucosamine sulfate slows down and reverses degeneration of cartilage within joints.

These studies are paramount in that no NSAID, including COX-2 inhibitors, have ever been able to retard the progression of osteoarthritis. Trials, which compared glucosamine sulfate to NSAIDS such as Ibuprofen, showed that long-term reductions in pain were greater in patients taking glucosamine sulfate. Moreover, long-term glucosamine administration does not elicit the potentially dangerous side effects associated with the use of NSAIDS.

It is believed that glucosamine sulfate supplementation is dangerous for diabetics. This is not true. Studies show that due to the low glycemic index, there are no adverse effects when used at the proper dose of 1500-3000 mg daily.

Enhancing the effects of glucosamine sulfate, the nutrient MSM (methylsulfonylmethane or dimethyl sulfone) is frequently included in supplements. This is known as "combination therapy." MSM is an organic, sulfur-containing compound that occurs naturally in a variety of fruits, vegetables, grains, and animals, including humans. MSM (2-8 grams daily) works to heal joints by acting as an anti-inflammatory to the joints and to inhibit pain impulses along nerve fibers. Besides helping arthritis sufferers, MSM can be of great benefit to those with bursitis, tendonitis and conditions such as tennis elbow and repetitive strain injury. MSM is a safe and non-toxic substance. Highlighted by the peer reviewed medical journal *Clinical Drug Investigations*, combination therapy has been shown to work even better and faster at reducing pain and swelling and in improving the functional ability of joints when compared to using glucosamine sulfate and MSM individually.

Offering further benefits from combination therapy, ginger has also been shown to have unprecedented success at treating and circumventing joint pain. Zingiber officinale (ginger root) has been shown to be a potent inhibitor of both prostaglandins (PGE2) and leukotrienes (LTB4). These (PGE2) prostaglandins and leukotrienes (LTB4) are ubiquitous substances that initiate and control cell and tissue responses involved in a myriad of physiological processes. These include platelet aggregation, and rennin release and inflammation. Their overproduction has been implicated in the pathophysiology of cardiovascular diseases, cancer and inflammatory diseases such as osteoarthritis. To circumvent the overproduction of prostaglandins (PGE2) and leukotrienes (LTB4) one could use Ginger.

The use of Ginger has been shown to lessen the pain associated with osteoarthritis. One study conducted by the Department of Environmental Medicine in Denmark showed that of 56 patients (2 with rheumatoid arthritis, 18 with osteoarthritis, and 10 with muscular discomfort) taking Zingiber officinale, 75% experienced relief in pain and swelling.[87]

Combination therapy with glucosamine sulfate, MSM, and Ginger for 4 to 6 months is America's answer to the growing number of people who suffer from osteoarthritis. In contrast to NSAIDS, such combination therapy is inexpensive and elicits no negative side effects. These substances, like water, are non-toxic.

[87] Pavelka, Karel. et al. "Glucosamine Sulfate Use and Delay of Progression of Knee Osteoarthritis." *Archives of Internal Medicine.* Vol 162, Oct 14, 2002.
Alternative Medicine Review. Volume 4, Number 3. 1999.
Müller-Fasbender H, et al. "Glucosamine sulfate compared to ibuprofen in osteoarthritis." *Osteo Cartilage.* 1994; 2: 61-69.
Scroggie DA, et al. "The effect of glucosamine-chondroitin supplementation on glycosylated hemoglobin levels in patients with type 2 diabetes mellitus." *Archives of Internal Medicine.* 2003; 163:1587-1590.
Singh Gurkirpal, MD, "Recent Considerations in Nonsteroidal Anti-Inflammatory Drug Gastropathy." *The American Journal of Medicine.* July 27, 1998, p. 31S.
Srivastava, KC. et al. "Ginger (Zingiber officianale) in rheumatism and musculoskeletal disorders." *Medical Hypotheses.* 1992 Dec;39(4):342-8.
Kiuchi, F. et al. "Inhibition of prostaglandin and leukotriene biosynthesis by gingerols and diarylheptanoids." *Chemical and Pharmaceutical Bulletin* (Tokyo). 1992 Feb;40(2):387-91.
Srivastava, KC. et al. "Ginger (Zingiber officianale) in rheumatism and musculoskeletal disorders." *Medical Hypotheses.* 1992 Dec;39(4):342-8.

Myth #5 – Nutritional Supplements (AKA Nutraceuticals) are Dangerous and Ineffective.

Fact: Nutritional supplements are essential to the basic processes of life and are the key to healthy living.

To circumvent FDA approved drug addiction and avoid becoming a casualty to them, it is imperative that we seek nutritional supplementation, sometimes called nutraceuticals, in order to attain better health. Unfortunately, this is becoming exceedingly difficult. To ensure that nutritional supplements do not tread on prescription drug turf, the "pharmaceutical powers that be" have implemented several methods of silencing the proper use of nutritional supplements, despite their profound benefit. In short, lobbying for stringent regulations on nutritional supplements limits access to not only nutraceuticals, but also to information about them. These regulations are often passed with the support of the people by hoodwinking them into thinking that they are necessary for their own protection. The reality is that once passed, the people lose access to valuable nutritional supplements and the same people who supported it grow ill. Meanwhile, the drug manufacturers who lobbied for the regulations successfully secure their lion's share of the profits by minimizing competition and profiting from the sickness that follows. Let's look at some specific examples of how nutritional supplements are silenced.

First, education on the proper use of nutritional substances in order to achieve good health was removed from the medical school curriculum over 80 years ago! As a result, most medical doctors are unable to advise anyone on the use of nutritional supplements for attaining better health and to treat various forms of disease. Their only training is in prescription drugs. This explains the reluctance of medical doctors to teach patients about natural alternatives, as they simply don't know about them. Few medical doctors will admit to this. Instead, they will simply shrug off nutritional supplements as ineffective or dangerous. Such statements are baseless. Of course, a select few medical doctors have become excellent advisors on proper use of nutraceuticals. This is through self-education.

By studying a bit of history or reading medical journals, medical doctors would be shocked to learn that the nutritional supplements they often criticize are the foundation of modern medicine, which they blindly embrace. The design of prescription drugs by organic chemists is guided by knowledge obtained from their plant –based predecessors, which are commonly sold as nutritional supplements. The difference being that the prescription drug is a single isolate whereas the nutritional supplement contains a multitude of active substances. Because of "synergy" obtained from the multitude of active ingredients, the nutritional supplement is often safer and more effective than its drug counterpart. This is a paradox that goes virtually unnoticed among the pharmaceutically biased medical community, as well as the general public.

Second, having successfully removed the study of nutritional substances for health from medical school curriculums, the FDA has stonewalled ALL nutritional supplement manufacturers from educating their clients on nutritional supplements. Namely, the FDA passed the Dietary Supplement Health and Education Act (DSHEA) to prohibit manufacturers in the supplement industry to market or claim that their products "cure, mitigate, treat, or prevent" any given disease or illness; instead, they can only make general statements about their products. As a result, nutritional supplements are marketed without scientific research and carry labels that are intentionally vague and misleading to consumers. Therefore, finding what nutritional supplements to take for any given illness has become close to impossible for the average health consumer.

Further, removing nutritional supplements from the reach of the public, DSHEA also gave the FDA the authority to remove any nutritional supplement from the market if it "proved" to be unsafe. Because of their broad definition of "unsafe" and because most anything, even water, is unsafe in large amounts, the FDA can now ban any nutritional supplement which poses as competition to their pharmaceutical partners. Ephedra is a perfect example (see chapter 9).

Third, making it harder to know the truth behind nutritional supplements, lobbying by the pharmaceutical industry has enabled the drug community to influence congress, the FDA and the media to set a negative tone on the use of nutritional supplementation for health and longevity in the popular media. More often than not, the tone is that natural alternatives to prescription drugs are not only ineffective, but also dangerous. Unable to distinguish between the truth and profit motives, the general public has turned away from nutrition while embracing drugs. This is the antithesis of health.

And finally, on the worldwide front, the World Trade Organization (WTO) is working rigorously to convince the nations of the world that ALL human beings require the EXACT same amount of nutrients and that anything above this amount is dangerous. Under the guise of protecting vitamin consumers, the WTO is using what is known as the CODEX ALIMENTARIUS COMMISION (CAC) to further restrict the free use of nutritional supplements within the USA and worldwide. Specifically, the CAC is setting "Guidelines for Vitamin and Mineral Food Supplements." These guidelines are much more restrictive than current USA regulations and will dictate to the USA which nutrients are deemed safe, the maximum and minimum amounts allowed in a product, and related packaging and labeling requirements. These guidelines set by CAC will supercede the FDA and any regulations that have been put in place to protect access to nutritional supplements within the USA.

Properly stated, Dr. Matthias Rath, MD, has emphatically asserted that CAC is a "threat to mankind" due to its potential to remove the majority of nutritional supplements from the public. In line with this, the director for International Advocates for Health Freedom (IAHF), John Hammell, has strived relentlessly to voice that the goal of the CAC is simply to monopolize the sale of dietary supplements worldwide by restricting high potency vitamins and making them available only by prescription.

Of course, the CAC stands firm in their conviction that these guidelines are for the safety of others. If safety were the priority, then the WTO could use the CAC to protect us from prescription drugs, which kill 100,000 people every year in the USA, instead of wasting time on nutritional supplements, which have killed less people than rabid squirrel attacks. To counter attack this assault on your health by the WTO, visit www.iahf.com and donate to their cause, as they are actively fighting nutrient "harmonization" in the courts.

Combined, the previously mentioned strategies have protected and will continue to protect the profits of the drug industry while limiting access to nutritional supplements. If not banned, safe and effective nutritional supplements and unpatentable compounds are simply ignored by government officials and the popular media. Examples include, but surely are not limited to: hydrazine sulfate, laetrile, GHB, glyoxylide, and krebiozen, just to name a few. Looking briefly at a few medicinal products that have proven health benefits but that are either banned or ignored better outlines how Americans are hoodwinked into thinking that nutritional supplements, which tread on pharmaceutical turf, are ineffective and unsafe.

Hydrazine sulfate (HS), discovered by biochemist Joseph Gold in 1968, is an unpatentable chemical that has been used successfully to stop cachexia (caKEKsia). Cachexia is a wasting process that occurs among cancer patients and AIDS patients. Cachexia kills 70% of cancer victims, but can be circumvented by the use of HS.[88] In addition to preventing the loss of body weight and body mass associated with cachexia, HS also stabilizes and reverses tumor growth without any toxic effects on healthy cells, making it an excellent anti-tumor agent and alternative to currently used chemotherapy drugs. The National Cancer Institute has identified studies where complete tumor regression was achieved among cancer patients who took HS.

These abilities of HS are derived from the fact that it blocks the production of excess glucose in the body, the primary fuel for cancer growth. When the glucose supply is cut

---

[88] Haley, Daniel. *Politics in Healing*. Potomac Valley Press. Copyright 2001. ISBN# 0-9701150-0-8.

off to cancer, it dies. Biochemists have found this ability of HS to be achieved from the inhibition of an enzyme known as PEP CK (phosphoenolpyruvate carboxykinase).

As early as 1976, adverse politics began taking its toll on HS. Due to poorly controlled scientific studies, courtesy of Sloan Kettering Institute, HS became known as ineffective, dangerous, and unsuitable for cancer treatment. Today, officials label HS as a cancer-causing substance while making it clear that the use of HS outside the context of clinical trials has not been approved by the Food and Drug Administration (FDA) and, thus, cannot be recommended. Interestingly, a 10-year supply of HS costs as much as one treatment of today's chemotherapy agents, which, as announced by Dr. Gold, can produce as much as 26% of "second cancers."

Further treading on conventional medicine's turf in the area of cancer treatment is an evergreen tree known as the Graviola tree. Native to South and North America, the Graviola tree produces an abundance of unpatentable chemicals known as acetogenins (*annonaceous acetogenins*). Acetogenins deplete cancer cells of their energy supply, adenosine triphosphate (ATP), thereby "unplugging" them from their life force, so to speak. Consequently, the cancer cell dies. Because healthy cells require much less ATP for survival, they remain alive during the ATP depletion. It is cancer's greediness for ATP that causes it to die while healthy cells remain alive once exposed to the acetogenins found in Graviola.

In addition to cancer, The NCI was among the first to discover that acetogenins had laser-like effectiveness at eradicating cancer cells that had become resistant to anti-cancer drugs, while leaving non-cancerous cells healthy. These findings were detailed in the *Journal of Medicinal Chemistry* and

Cancer Letters.[89] Scientists from around the world have been following up on this research ever since. As recent as 2003, scientist Nakanishi and colleagues from University of North Carolina at Chapel Hill discovered several acetogenins from Graviola that selectively killed ovarian cancer cells.[90] Looking at other forms of cancer, scientists Wang and colleagues from Toyama Medical and Pharmaceutical University found that acetogenins were also deadly to lung cancer.[91] The National Cancer Institute (NCI) began screening acetogenins in an attempt to synthesize (make in a lab) derivatives (other forms) and patent them for profit. Due to their complex structures, many labs have simply given up on making derivatives of these compounds. Therefore, Graviola has been pushed under the pharmaceutical rug, thereby shielding it from public knowledge.

Green Tea Extract (GTE), contains natural compounds known as catechins (also known as polyphenols), and is repeatedly showing anti-cancer benefits as well. That these benefits are being proven time and again around the world warrants massive media coverage. Recent studies show that a synergistic blend of 8 catechins from GTE reduces breast tumor volume almost 10 fold and overall tumor inhibition by 80-90%.[92] Chemotherapy drugs approved by the FDA pale

---

[89] Oberlies, NH. et al. "The annonaceous acetogenins bullaticin is cytotoxic against multidrug-resistant human mammary adenocarcinoma cells." *Cancer Letters.* 1997 May 1;115(1):73-9.

[90] Nakanishi Y. et al. "Acetogenins as selective inhibitors of the human ovarian 1A9 tumor cell line." *Journal of Medical Chemistry.* 2003 Jul 17;46(15):3185-8.

[91] Wang LQ. Et al. "Annonaceous acetogenins from the leaves of Annona Montana." Bioorganic and Medicinal Chemistry. 2002 Mar;10(3):561-5.

[92] *Nutrition and Cancer.* 2001;40(2);149-56.
Phytotherapy Research. 2002 Mar; 16 Suppl 1:S40-4.
British Journal of Cancer. 2002 May 20;86(10);1645-51.

in comparison to isolated compounds from green tea. GTE is non-toxic both in acute dosage and high long-term dosage. Unlike currently approved chemotherapy drugs, GTE has no potential for causing mutations or birth defects, and has no adverse effect on fertility, pregnancy or nursing.

In addition to fighting cancer and being non-toxic, GTE acts as an antioxidant, lowers serum glucose (thereby working to prevent insulin resistance and type II diabetes), maintains kidney health, and prevents clot formation. Other studies are showing that GTE can prevent, and possibly treat, numerous other diseases including arthritis, stroke and cardiovascular disease. Just recently, GTE was shown to prevent high blood pressure by up to 65% among habitual (one year of use) users, as reported in the *Archives of Internal Medicine.*[93]

With all certainty, a proper extract of green tea catechins would be among the most potent nutritional supplements on the planet and would play an integral role in increasing longevity if taken once daily. If a synthetic drug had half the potential of wiping out common afflictions akin to GTE it would be considered the latest "wonder drug" and your doc would be throwing samples in the street, as they do with Vioxx and Lipitor.

Whey protein isolate is another excellent example of a safe and effective cancer fighter that is rarely discussed. In the hunt for natural anti-cancer drugs, researchers have found that whey isolate delivers a unique cancer-fighting protein known as lactoferrin to the body. Secondly, through a process known as "conjugation," whey isolate also helps to rid the body of cancer causing substances, known as carcinogens, by attaching to them and escorting them out of the body and into the toilet.

---

[93] *Archives of Internal Medicine* 164, 14:1534-1540, 2004.

Evidence for whey's cancer preventing and fighting ability has been documented in *Anticancer Research and Cancer Letters*. When referring to whey isolate, scientists have emphatically stated, "this non-toxic dietary intervention, which is not based on the principles of current cancer chemotherapy, will hopefully attract the attention of laboratory and clinical oncologists."[94]

Substantiating the cancer fighting ability of whey isolate, *Cancer Letters* stated: "Epidemiological and experimental studies suggest that dietary milk products [such as whey] may exert an inhibitory effect on the development of several tumors."[95] Enthusiastic researchers at the Department of Food Science & Technology at Ohio State University demonstrated that the active protein in whey isolate, lactoferrin, increased glutathione levels in prostate cells by 50%, thereby significantly preventing prostate cancer.[96] Researchers at Lund University in Sweden reported that the use of whey in combination with an unnamed component of human breast milk, have demonstrated the ability to kill all known types of breast cancer cells. Their peer-reviewed paper, published in the *Journal of Biological Chemistry*, suggested that when consumed by the body, whey proteins selectively induce "programmed cell death," AKA suicide, among breast cancer tumors.[97] This is known scientifically as apoptosis.

---

[94]   *Anticancer Research.* 2000 Nov-Dec;20(6C);4785-92.

[95]   *Cancer Letters.* 1991 May 1;57(2):91-4.

[96]   K. D. Kent. et al. Dept. of Food Science and Technology, Ohio State Univ. 2002.

[97]   Journal of Biological Chemistry. 274:6388-6396, 1999.

Shane Ellison M.Sc.

Smoothie for Maximizing Childhood Health and Development

The following smoothie recipe is designed to not only taste good but also provide children with essential nutrients for proper development, immune boosting, cognitive enhancement well being. Parents will see the difference.

Whey Advanced (www.health-fx.net) can be blended into a great tasting "smoothie." This is a great option for children (for breakfast or lunch), those looking for a great tasting snack and also athletes who need either a pre or post event carbo/protein meal.

Place in a blender or food processor and blend until smooth:

4 ounces of organic orange juice

6 ounces of water

1-5 g of Blue-Green Algae

1 banana

3 whole strawberries (frozen)

3 ice cubes

1 scoop of Whey Advanced (3 tablespoons)

Scientists in Japan announced that lactoferrin (from whey isolate) significantly inhibits colon, esophagus, lung, bladder and tongue cancer in animal models.[98] And last but not least, there is very strong evidence that whey proteins render cancerous cells more vulnerable to chemotherapy and radiation while protecting healthy cells from their devastating side effects! But unlike chemotherapy and ionizing radiation, whey

---

[98]   Foods Food Ingredients Journal of Japan No. 200 (2002).

proteins have no toxic side affects. Whey literally does the patient no harm.

Last but not least, the most entertaining of all the unpatentable nutrients that have been shown to have anti-cancer effects is GHB (gamma-hydroxy butyrate). In an attempt to increase the oral availability of the neurotransmitter GABA, Henri Laborit first made GHB, a naturally occurring GABA derivative, as early as the 1960's. Markedly, this allowed the GABA derivative to sail directly into the blood stream and penetrate the often hard to pass blood-brain barrier when consumed orally. Further, it was found that GHB was absolutely non-toxic, as it was metabolized into CO_2 and water! Therefore, it does not cause any adverse effects to organs of the body. At this point, GHB became the center of study worldwide. Most notably, scientists found that GHB significantly suppressed tumor growth due to its ability to inhibit angiogenesis. Among cancer patients, GHB was able to increase 5-year survival rates by a whopping 20.7%. This is considerably better than the oft-prescribed cancer drug cisplatin. That it is non-toxic puts it light years ahead of currently prescribed chemotherapy drugs.

Slowly but surely, GHB received worldwide notoriety among the public, but not for its positive effects. Instead, because excess GHB can cause users to pass out (like alcohol but without damage to liver), it was labeled the date rape drug by the FDA and considered lethal even in small quantities. Apparently, they failed to check with the Drug Enforcement Agency (DEA) who reported a mere 58 deaths over a period of 10 years from GHB use, most likely due to improper use among unhealthy individuals. Regardless, using the hysteria brought about by the media as momentum, the US government quickly outlawed GHB with the passing of the Hillory J. Farias and Samantha Reid Date-Rape Drug Prohibition Act of 2000. Officially, this made GHB a schedule I drug in the United States.

Not being able to patent GHB for profit, but recognizing its benefits as an anti-cancer drug, chemists from Bristol Myers Squibb got creative by designing a "pro-drug" to GHB, named UFT (Uracil-tegafur). Once consumed, UFT is converted into GHB. Because UFT is man made, it was patented and is now used extensively in Asia, Europe, and Latin America. In the Unites States, however, the FDA has refused to approve UFT. Commenting on why the FDA has refused approval, Dr. Herman Kattlove of Los Angeles, medical editor for the American Cancer Society (ACS), has stated "finding a drug as simple as this, as free of side effects, that works is just too good to be true."[99]

Relative to the parent drug, UFT has inherent downfalls compared to GHB. This is mostly due to the unknown effects of two other metabolites of UFT, known as GBL and 5-FU. Using GHB directly is far safer and obviously less expensive than the man-made drug UFT. Recognizing this, the FDA has quietly assured a small drug company, Orphan Medical Inc. that GHB is safe for use and has allowed them to distribute GHB legally under the trade name Xyrem. In addition to being offered 7-year exclusivity (monopoly) on this unpatentable compound, Orphan Medical, Inc. is allowed to charge 20X the street value for GHB while at the same time receive tax credit for product-associated clinical research of GHB.

A most important note is the aforementioned exciting nature of GHB. GHB elicits unequivocal euphoria among users, without causing any hangover or toxic effects. When used properly, GHB could be considered the Holy Grail for

---

[99] "Drug combo may help slow lung cancer." Study on FDA-rejected treatment surprises U.S. experts. *The Associated Press.* Updated: 3:53 p.m. ET April 21, 2004.

unleashing dormant feelings of happiness, love and even lust; something the world could use a lot more of. The ability of GHB gives rise to its use in curing alcoholism and drug addiction as well as severe cases of depression. Users of GHB are also rewarded with a surge in Human Growth Hormone (hGH) levels, thereby making it a novel anti-aging nutrient.

To date, it appears that this non-toxic alternative to chemotherapy is gone forever, while alcohol, which kills 100,000 per year, remains on the shelves as the number one date-rape drug of all time. Way to go parents! Perhaps when their children suffer from cancer, they can wish them a good farewell with a cold beer rather than providing them with GHB to increase their chance of being cured by 20%. No doubt, they will then take note of their error of supporting the illegalization of GHB, instigated by lazy reporting and egregiously false implications by the FDA.

Of particular importance to the elderly and endurance athletes are the nutritional supplements acetyl-L-carnitine (ALCAR) (not L-carnitine) and alpha-lipoic acid (ALA). Their modes of action within our bodies, being extremely complex, provide an entire array of health benefits.

The use of ALCAR increases energy production within the body and the biosynthesis of the brain neurotransmitter acetylcholine. This translates into the prevention and retardation of Alzheimer's Disease (AD), Parkinson's Disease and geriatric depression, as outlined by Pettegrew and colleagues from University of Pittsburg and published in *Molecular Psychiatry*.[100]

Those who suffer from Multiple Sclerosis (MS) also benefit from ALCAR supplementation. Researchers Tomassini and colleagues from the University of Rome show that ALCAR

---

[100] Pettegrew, et al. *Molecular Psychiatry* . (2000) 5, 616-632.

increases energy levels among sufferers of MS more effectively than the commonly prescribed drug for treating MS, amantadine.[101]

Those with a broken heart, or who fear a broken heart, will be happy to hear that ALCAR is a solid mend. Lonnis Rizos of the University of Athens Medical School documented a 15% decrease in absolute mortality rates among those patients who suffered from heart failure and subsequently supplemented with ALCAR for 3 years.[102] Scientists Cavallini and colleagues show that, like androgen administration, ALCAR proved to be an effective drug for the therapy of symptoms associated with male aging, but without the negative side effects often seen among users of androgens (AKA steroids).[103] Administration of ALCAR among the elderly results in a reduction of total fat mass and an increase in total muscle mass.

An important observation, ALCAR surpasses the metabolic potency of carnitine because it is a source of the precious acetyl group. The acetyl group facilitates energetic pathways which carnitine cannot supply. For the technical mind, acetyl groups from ALCAR can be combined with coenzyme A (the metabolized form of the vitamin pantothenic acid) to create Acetyl-Coenzyme A (A-CoA). A-CoA, acting within the Krebs cycle, helps generate the energy-producing molecule ATP. Lacking the acetyl group, there is little chance that L-carnitine can enhance ATP production, unless it picks up acetyl groups in the bloodstream. Because ALCAR already carries the acetyl group, use of it over L-carnitine culminates in greater energy production among all cells of the body as reported by the School of Medicine at the University of Sienna.[104]

---

[101] Tomassini, V. et al. *Journal of Neurological Science.* 2004 Mar 15;218(1-2):103-8.

[102] Rizos Ionnis. *American Heart Journal.* Volume 139, Number 2, Part 3.

[103] Cavallini G, et al. *Urology.* 2004 Apr; 63(4):641-6.

[104] Capecchi PL, et al. *Vascular Medicine.* 1997;2(2):77-81.

Noting that ALCAR uses enhances ATP, the implications for athletes who thrive on ATP are obvious. Supplementation with ALCAR leads to an increase in the strength of muscle contractions as well as shortened recovery times and increased endurance. It is estimated that endurance athletes can only obtain 300 mg of ALCAR from diet, yet they require 3,000 to 4,000 mg per day for optimal performance. Clearly, supplemented athletes would gain a significant advantage over their non-supplemented competitors.

Alpha lipoic acid (ALA) has been considered the Master antioxidant. It is unique in that, unlike any other antioxidant, ALA is both fat and water soluble; thereby allowing it to operate in all environments in the body. Moreover, ALA inhibits the "hydroxyl radical." The hydroxyl radical is considered to be the most damaging of the free radicals due to its ability to initiate "lipoprotein peroxidation." Lipoprotein peroxidation can lead to the much talked about and dangerous "oxidized LDL molecule." This is of paramount importance in that if the hydroxyl radical is not inhibited, then the "oxidized LDL molecule" might cause undesirable health problems such as atherosclerosis, which leads to heart disease.

Adding to the myriad of benefits, ALA regenerates (through redox cycling) other antioxidants like vitamin C and vitamin E, thus helping to prevent a deficiency in any one of these vital nutrients. This alone prevents a laundry list of known illnesses caused by deficiencies in C and E, most notably heart disease.

ALA also maintains and even increases our bodies' own antioxidant: glutathione. Glutathione's best attribute is its ability to protect us from cancer; therefore, any increase is greatly warranted and benefited from. Glutathione is the chief detoxifier for the human body. Through a process known as "conjugation" it attaches to deadly chemicals and escorts them out of the body and into the toilet. No other antioxidant has this ability.

ALA is crucial for diabetics. ALA has been used for approximately 30 years in Europe to treat diabetic neuropathy, regulate blood sugar and prevent diabetic retinopathy and weakening of the heart.

Using ALCAR and ALA together increases ones chances of maximizing functional life span. Highlighted in the *Proceedings of the National Academy of Sciences*, Bruce Ames and colleagues state that using these essential nutrients may reverse the effects of aging on the brain. In 2003, *Reader's Digest* referred to the combined use of ALA and ALCAR as the "Pill that can end aging."

Nutritional supplementation in children also provides immeasurable benefits. Zinc supplementation given to nutrient-starved children in Bangladeshi prevented absolute death by 50% and decreased the need for antibiotics by 60% among those who suffered from diarrhea.[105] Typically, 20 mg of elemental zinc was administered daily for 14 days during each episode of diarrhea. Lead author Abdullah Baqui, MBBS, MPH, DrPH, Associate Professor of International Health at the Johns Hopkins Bloomberg School of Public Health explains, "The lower rates of child morbidity and mortality with zinc therapy represent substantial benefits from a simple and inexpensive intervention. Zinc can be incorporated within existing diarrheal disease control efforts, which should significantly improve child health and survival."

Zinc also affords children a 41% reduction in pneumonia. Reported in the *Journal of Pediatric* and written by scientists

---

[105] Abdullah H Baqui, et al. "Effect of zinc supplementation started during diarrhoea on morbidity and mortality in Bangladeshi children: community randomised trial." *British Medical Journal.* 2002; 325: 1059.

from the Johns Hopkins School of Health, the sum effect of zinc supplementation on childhood health has a greater preventative effect for pneumonia, which kills millions of children per year, than any other current intervention. Such results often go ignored, and instead of nutritional supplements, children are often administered mass vaccination under the auspices of "charity work" by drug companies. True charity would be the administration of nutritional supplements that, like zinc, increase survival rates by 50%. Of course, drug companies would have to take a 60% loss in antibiotic use.

There's more good news for children: Expecting and nursing mothers who supplement with Vitamin A (beta-carotene) can lower their children's risk of death by up to 40% compared to mothers who do not supplement Vitamin A. This discovery was made looking at women in south rural Asia, who have a mortality rate 50 to 100 times higher than in industrialized countries. Death usually results from severe bleeding, obstructed labor, infection and Vitamin A deficiency. Take note, though, you wont see any news sources showing wanna-be philanthropic drug companies offering Vitamin A to rural villages. Not in this lifetime.

This is an extremely short list of safe and beneficial nutritional supplements. New safe and effective nutritional supplements are being discovered almost daily. Despite the short list herein, it would appear that when put toe-to-toe against FDA approved drugs, the benefits derived from these few nutritional supplements exceeds all of those obtained from the entire array of FDA approved drugs; outside of emergency medicine, of course. To validate this, simply look at the enormous amount of prescription drugs being used in the United States, the extreme lack of health in the Unites States and the

Shane Ellison M.Sc.

100,000 plus people who die every year in the United States from FDA approved drugs.[106]

To assert that nutritional supplements are ineffective and unsafe while praising FDA approved drugs borders lunacy. This lunacy is easy to explain. As a contributing editor to the *Journal of Orthomolecular Medicine*, Andrew Saul, PhD, tells us that:

> "I have learned that it is easier for most researchers to get a negative vitamin study published [in a peer reviewed medical journal] than a positive one. As with the evening news, where the policy is usually 'If it bleeds, it leads,' the scare story sells. Same with vitamin articles: the shock-story gets the front page. There is some strong economic inertia at work. Successful vitamin therapy is a triple threat to the medical cartel. It threatens physicians because they know practically nothing about it, and it represents real competition. It threatens the pharmaceutical industry because vitamins cannot be patented and sold at huge profits. It threatens dieticians because the fallaciousness of their food-groups-always, supplements-never dogma will be exposed. In all three cases, it is the very success of vitamin therapy that is cause for such alarm."

It appears that such lunacy has led many Americans to deny nutritional supplementation. According to the National Center for Health Statistics, only nine percent of all American adults consume enough healthy foods to reach their minimum recommended daily intake of nutrients to assure proper health. This translates into a massive nutrient deficit among Americans. To be precise, 90% of American adults lack es-

[106] Lucian Leape, "Error in medicine." *Journal of the American Medical Association.* 1994, 272:23, p 1851. Also: Leape LL. "Institute of Medicine medical error figures are not exaggerated." *Journal of the American Medical Association.* 2000 Jul 5;284(1):95-7.

sential nutrients to stay alive. It would not be a stretch to say that this 90% is slowly dying. Johns Hopkins Medical School, who published the studies of Ames and Wakimoto, has clarified this. These researchers found that "suboptimal nutrient intake is a widespread problem."[107] Such nutrients include, but are not limited to, vitamin C, folic acid, magnesium, acetyl-L-carnitine, bioactive peptides, zinc, copper, B12, essential fatty acids, vitamin D and selenium.

The importance of these nutrients demands attention. Take heed. A lack of nutrients results in a lack of "metabolic harmony." Metabolic harmony can be described as the ability of your body to properly maintain DNA function by minimizing damage to DNA. DNA serves as a genetic map, continually working to guide your body to proper health. A deficiency in any ONE nutrient can wreak havoc on DNA, thereby disrupting the mechanism by which DNA directs the body to perfect health. The result is the loss of function in many systems of the body. For instance, as noted by Ames and Wakimoto, a single deficiency can lead to cancer (pancreatic, bone, prostate, etc.), premature aging (aching joints, low hormone levels, Parkinson's, wrinkled skin, etc.) and loss of mental function (Alzheimer's, etc.) due to increased damage to DNA from a nutritional deficiency.

This explains how many nutrients afford users so many different health benefits.

Indirectly, burying or subverting the use of nutritional alternatives to drugs has killed millions who would have otherwise led healthy lives from the use of them. Boldly stated, the Centers for Disease Control (CDC) explains that, combined, unhealthy eating [not obtaining essential nutrients] and physi-

[107] Ames, Bruce. Wakimoto, Patricia. "Are Vitamin Deficiencies a Major Caner Risk?" 2002 *Nature Publishing Group*. September. Volume 2.

cal inactivity contributes to at least 400,000 deaths every year, which equates to 4 million every 10 years. Offering hints as to how to prevent this tragedy, the CDC reports that the chronic disease burden now plaguing America would be entirely preventable if we simply changed our eating habits to include vital nutrients (via diet or nutritional supplementation).

In addition to saving lives, nutritional supplementation would save money. A study by The Lewin Group estimated the potential economic savings to the Medicare system that might be afforded by the use of daily multivitamin supplements among seniors (65 years and older) in the United States. For a five-year period (2004-2008), the figure was estimated to be as much as $1.6 billion. This study was based on an analysis of various types of studies, including randomized clinical trials, cohort studies, case control studies, cross-sectional studies, and using Congressional Budget Office accounting methods. The Lewin Group study concluded that multivitamin use may considerably decrease hospitalizations and nursing home care for heart disease and infections. For instance, one study highlighted by the Lewin Group involved 80,000 nurses and found a 24 percent reduction in the risk of heart attacks among women who took daily multivitamins. Of course, medical doctors would be forced to take huge pay cuts along with drug companies.

Prevention could not get any easier. Taking nutritional supplements via food or in a capsule requires no large expense, no doctor's appointment and no physical work whatsoever. It is the American Dream, being healthy without doing anything! This reminds me of the acronym KISS. Perhaps our self-appointed medical authorities should be reminded of it in order to help Americans regain their health: Keep It Simple Stupid.

It's important to realize that the use of nutritional supplements varies considerably among individuals. Using nutritional supplements to heal various forms of disease can be a complex matter. To say that one single nutritional supplement (or FDA approved drug for that matter) is good for everyone is saying that all humans are created equal. This is simply not true.

Using nutritional supplements for procuring good health is not as easy as taking a recommended dosage of a given substance. Of great importance is the purity of the extract (when applicable), the proper dose relative to weight and age, the correct time of day to take it, understanding whether or not there are dangerous interactions with other foods, and knowing how long the treatment should last. For instance, Graviola cannot be taken with the commonly used nutrient known as CoQ10. CoQ10 works to upregulate the production of ATP, while Graviola works to downregulate its production. Taken together they cancel each other out and become ineffective. Additionally, Graviola cannot be taken for long periods of time due to its overall affect on slowing ATP production. If taken for a long period of time, users may become overtly fatigued. Another striking example of negative interaction would be using whey isolate with sugar or sugar alternatives, because these added ingredients would contribute to cancer while canceling the beneficial effects of whey isolate. Because of these many considerations, it is imperative that you do your research or consult with a knowledgeable source before moving forward.

To aid in the pursuit of safe and effective natural medicine, the members' section at www.healthmyths.net will provide a "nutritional supplement review." Owners of this book can access using the password "naturalhealth."

The underlying message is that pharmaceutical drugs simply impersonate science while nutraceuticals embrace it.

You see, pharmaceutical drugs have ZERO value outside of an EMERGENCY and are obsolete based on current scientific research. This is why the pharmaceutical industry has to design and fund their own studies while being forced to spend billions of dollars on drug marketing in order to sell these poisons. Those who rely on this medical model for health are going against scientific reality. This would be akin to asserting that the world is flat to a sailor who had successfully traveled around the globe. Other false medical models include taking cholesterol-lowering drugs to prevent heart disease, using prescription drugs to prevent obesity, administering stimulants such as Ritalin or Adderall to treat ADHD, consuming selective serotonin reuptake inhibitors (SSRI's) like Prozac to treat depression and vaccinating to prevent disease. These treatments, in the long run, are worse then the so-called disease.

Despite the advances made in the study of nutrition, not a single one of the mentioned nutrients in this chapter are FDA approved. Thanks to the US government's passing of DSHEA, manufacturers of the nutrition supplements are not allowed to highlight their benefits in their marketing material. Understanding the benefits of nutritional supplements, and the US government's unwillingness to acknowledge them, helps us better understand the one-sided health model that is adhered to in the United States simply for the reason of wealth, not health.

In order to overcome these obstacles, consumers must become educated on the facts and understand the implications of both nutritional supplement use and the use of FDA approved drugs. This will allow for a free market based on knowledge where non-toxic therapies can compete freely with the toxic therapies that ultimately hinder basic human development.

Optimal health results from a balance of science and nature. Unfortunately, "cookie-cutter doctors" and the "pharmaceutically correct FDA" have abandoned both and reached for profits. Consequently, most people have become victims of health fascism rather than health freedom.

Myth #6 - High Cholesterol is a Major Risk Factor for Heart Disease

Fact: High blood cholesterol is not a major contributing factor to heart disease.

The assertion that high cholesterol is a major risk factor for heart disease is the biggest health myth of all time. As such, this chapter will be hotly debated and will threaten the reputations of leading health practitioners and pharmaceutical companies worldwide. Regardless, the truth speaks for itself.

For the record, heart disease, the leading cause of death for all Americans aged 35 and older, is clinically defined as the narrowing or hardening of the arteries. Arteries are large blood vessels that transport the blood away from the heart to various organs in the body. This transportation ensures that oxygen and nutrients are delivered to all areas of the body. Heart disease is often referred to as atherosclerosis. But in reality, atherosclerosis is the name of the process in which deposits of fatty substances, cholesterol, cellular waste products, white blood cells, calcium and other debris builds up in the inner lining of an artery. This buildup is called plaque and is the most common cause of heart disease. To reiterate, heart disease is often caused by atherosclerosis, which blocks arteries and results in a heart attack or stroke.

Rarely, if at all, is the definition or cause of heart disease explained. Instead, pharmaceutical giants and medical doctors repeatedly tell Americans that cholesterol must be lowered to prevent this pandemic killer. In the same breath, they offer cholesterol-lowering drugs. This 2-minute rendition is the extent of the treatment.

This dogma is well entrenched in the minds of professionals and laymen alike. To be exact, it is highly touted by the American Heart Association (AHA), who states that: "High blood cholesterol is a major risk factor for coronary heart disease and stroke." Medical evidence acquired over the last 100 years disproves this myth faster than a doctor can prescribe Lipitor.

Looking at trends among those with atherosclerosis and setting the following criteria can easily test the validity of the claim that "lowering cholesterol prevents heart disease." This criterion is a simple matter of action and reaction.

The myth is only true if there is a correlation between total cholesterol levels and the changes in atherosclerosis development.[108] In other words, as cholesterol increases, so should plaque within the arterial walls. Or as cholesterol decreases, so should atherosclerosis.

While this seems very trivial, few professionals are looking for this correlation to support their assertion that lowering cholesterol prevents heart disease.

---

[108] Ravnskov, U. "Is atherosclerosis caused by high cholesterol?" *Quarterly Journal of Medicine.* 2002; 95: 397-403.

Having set the criteria for testing the validity of the cholesterol myth, let us look at what the scientific method has shown to date with relation to cholesterol and atherosclerosis, the main culprit in heart disease.

Looking for a correlation between total cholesterol levels and the changes in atherosclerosis development, we must go all the way back to a landmark study from 1961. Researchers Mathur and colleagues studied the levels of cholesterol and the degree of atherosclerosis seen at autopsy within the arteries of 20 deceased patients as well as 200 more cases selected from medical libraries. All cholesterol levels were taken within 16 hours of death. Combined, no correlation could be observed between these patients' blood cholesterol levels and the amount or severity of "atherosclerotic plaque" within the arteries. Hence, cholesterol levels, whether high or low, had no impact on the growth of atherosclerotic plaque, the major cause of heart disease.[109] This study showed the exact opposite of what Americans are told and shakes the very foundation of the current medical model for treating or preventing heart disease.

Many other studies have confirmed these findings by Mathur and colleagues. *The American Journal of Clinical Nutrition* has also shown that at autopsy, postmortem patients who died suddenly showed no correlation between total cholesterol levels and atherosclerosis. In their research, Jose Mendez, PhD, and co-workers point out that their findings agree with previous studies. Notably, they cited researchers Lande and Sperry who in 1936 also failed to find a correlation between cholesterol levels and atherosclerotic plaque.[110]

---

[109] Mathur, K.S. et al. "Serum Cholesterol and Atherosclerosis in Man." *Circulation.* 1961:23:847-52.

[110] Lande, et al. "Human atherosclerosis in relation to the cholesterol content of blood serum." *Archives of Pathology.* 22:301, 1936.

Looking at further evidence, in 1962, the *American Heart Journal* published the research of Dr. Marek and colleagues who, among 106 cases studied, also found that the level of cholesterol does not affect atherosclerotic changes in plaque.[111] Dr. Marek concluded by stating that his results do not differ from the results obtained under the exact same examinations in health and disease with atherosclerosis, conducted by the same methods, in the same laboratory, and in the same populations.

Decades of research failed to find any correlation between atherosclerosis and cholesterol levels. Because the entire medical community, and the world for that matter, asserts that there is a correlation between atherosclerosis and cholesterol, we forge ahead by looking for proof.

Continuing the search for a correlation between cholesterol levels and atherosclerotic plaque buildup, we can use state of the art technology. Rather than looking at arteries before and after death we can simply look at them while the patient is alive. More specifically, we can utilize a special X-ray imaging machine, known as electron beam computed tomography (EBCT), to look at both cholesterol levels and atherosclerosis buildup in the arteries without waiting for patients to die. Electron beam tomography represents the next level in cardiac diagnosis by allowing medical doctors to visualize the coronary arteries without having to go through an invasive procedure.

Utilizing EBCT technology, researchers Hecht and Harman of Beth Israel Medical Center in New York set out to determine whether or not increased cholesterol levels, specifically LDL cholesterol, led to plaque build up. Looking at 182 individuals who may develop symptoms of heart disease over

---

[111] Marek, et al. "Atherosclerosis and levels of serum cholesterol in post mortem investigation." *American Heart Journal.* 1962.

1.2 years of treatments with cholesterol lowering drugs alone or in combination with niacin, it was discovered that despite lower cholesterol levels, there were ZERO differences in the development of atherosclerotic plaque. These researchers concluded, "with respect to LDL cholesterol lowering, "lower is better" is not supported by changes in calcified plaque progression."[112] Not surprisingly, as noted by CNN, medical doctors and drug companies who circulate the cholesterol myth are threatened by EBCT. [113]

Unable to find any evidence to support the cholesterol lowering myth, we can turn the pages in our history books. Extrapolating data from history, if high cholesterol was the culprit in heart disease, then earlier cholesterol lowering drugs known as "fibrates" would have prevented deaths form heart disease. Yet, this was not the case! In their report to congress, entitled *Cholesterol Treatment – A Review of the Clinical Trials Evidence*, the US General Accounting Office (GAO) stated, "With respect to total fatalities—that is, deaths from CHD [heart disease] and all other causes—most meta-analyses show no significant difference and thus no improvement in overall survival rates in the trials [using fibrates] that included either persons with known CHD or persons without it."

Recognizing that drug companies and purveyors of the cholesterol myth would not be happy with this conclusion, the GAO finished by recognizing that "This finding, that cholesterol treatment has not lowered the number of deaths over-

[112] Hecht HS, Harmann SM. "Relation of aggressiveness of lipid-lowering treatment to changes in calcified plaque burden by electron beam tomography." *American Journal of Cardiology.* 2003 Aug 1;92(3):334-6.
[113] http://www.cnn.com/HEALTH/library/HB/00015.html.

all, has been worrisome to many researchers and is at the core of much of the controversy on cholesterol policy."[114]

Further, to find more evidence to determine whether or not high cholesterol has an impact on atherosclerosis we can use the highly touted "statin drug trials." These were well-funded studies, looking at the effects of the newer generation cholesterol lowering drugs, statins, on atherosclerosis.

If high cholesterol were the cause of heart disease, then the greatest preventative effects from statin drugs would be seen among those with the highest cholesterol levels and in patients whose cholesterol levels were lowered the most. This has yet to be seen in any study.[115]

Looking at the statin drug trial known as the Heart Protection Study (HPS) and the Scandinavian Simvastatin Survival Study (4s), statin drugs are just as effective whether cholesterol is lowered by a small amount or by more than 40%. For instance, the same benefits from Zocor were seen in patients who had a 40% drop in cholesterol and who had no drop in cholesterol! Scientists recognizing this stated, "Surprisingly, people [using Zocor (simvastatin)] in the Study [HPS] with normal or low cholesterol had the same heart benefits as those with high cholesterol."[116, 117]

To highlight this point, we can look to the latest and greatest statin drug Crestor. Crestor plummeted cholesterol levels,

---

[114] US General Accounting Office. "Cholesterol Treatment. A Review of the Clinical Evidence." 1996.

[115] Ravnskov U. "High cholesterol may protect against infections and atherosclerosis." *Quarterly Journal of Medicine.* 2003;96:927-34.

[116] http://www.zocor.com/simvastatin/zocor/consumer/have_a_prescription_for_zocor/zocor_helps_reduce_risk.jsp

[117] Ravnskov, Uffe. "High Cholesterol may Protect against Infection and Atherosclerosis."

yet failed to show any effectiveness, as could be seen by a 0% decrease in total mortality rates among users.

Other drugs show this same tendency. A drug trial known as REVERSAL showed that while Pravachol lowered LDL cholesterol by 25% it failed to stop the progression of heart disease, as could be seen by the continued growth of atheroma (thickening and fatty degeneration of the inner coat of the arteries).[118] Lead investigator, Dr. Steven Nissen, was dumb-founded and commented that:

> "Surprisingly, despite attaining a low LDL level on pravas-tatin [Pravachol], these patients showed highly significant progression for percent atheroma volume and percent obstructive volume..."

He continued by saying:

> "When I started this study, I believed that any reduction in progression would just be due to lower LDL levels, but now I'm not so sure."

Admittedly, researchers have shown statin treatment to be effective in high-risk individuals who showed lower cholesterol from the use of the drugs. However, confidently speaking, this is not due to their cholesterol lowering effect. Simply, such benefits derived from statins are due to a direct drug effect rather than the side effect of lowering cholesterol. It is almost as if drug companies recognized this and instead of remedying the negative side effect, simply brow beat Americans into thinking it was a good thing.

That statin benefits are not attributed to their ability to drastically lower cholesterol is not inexplicable. Heart disease has

---

[118] Hughes, Sue. "REVERSAL: Atorvastatin 80 mg halts atheroma progression, pravastatin 40 mg does not." *Heart Wire*. November 13, 2003. Copyright ©1999 - 2003 theheart.org.

many features of an "inflammatory disease" (as you will learn in the next chapter). In fact, lesions within the arterial lining (endothelium) contain inflammatory cells. Therefore, any nutrient or drug that carried with it anti-inflammatory properties would inhibit their growth of plaque, thereby slowing or stopping the progression of heart disease. Scientist Marz and colleagues from the Karl Franzens University in Austria have shown in their lab that statin drugs do in fact have anti-inflammatory actions on cells within the arteries.[119] Therefore, it is scientifically sound to hypothesize that the direct drug effect of statins is related to anti-inflammation, not cholesterol lowering.

Not to get sidetracked from the cholesterol issue, let's briefly look closer at inflammation. The inflammatory response associated with heart disease is induced by damage to the inner lining of the artery. This damage activates the immune system, which in turn begins to initiate a complex inflammatory cascade leading to the formation of "foam cells" (a biomarker for this process is C-reactive protein). The formation and accumulation of foam cells is the first manifestation of plaque and is mainly due to "sticky" proteins called cellular adhesion molecules. These molecules, like bubble gum sticking to the bottom of a desk, adhere to the surface of damaged arterial lining. The nutrient alpha-lipoic acid (ALA) has been shown to block these "sticky" proteins, cellular adhesion molecules.[120] By doing so, ALA use can prevent excess plaque buildup. Unlike statin drugs, ALA has no negative side effects.

Showing more promise than vitamin C and the body's natural antioxidant, glutathione (this however, is not to discount

[119] Marz, W. et al. "HMG-CoA reductase inhibition: anti-inflammatory effects beyond lipid lowering?" *Journal of Cardiovascular Risk.* 2003 Jun;10(3):169-79.
[120] Zhang, W.J. and Frei, B. (2001) "Alpha-lipoic acid inhibits TNF-alpha-induced NF-kappaB activation and adhesion molecule expression in human aortic endothelial cells." *FASEB Journal.* 15:2423-2432.

the use of vitamin C or the importance of glutathione, as they play crucial biological roles outside of anti-inflammation), ALA has proven to be an effective anti-inflammatory agent for the prevention of heart disease.[121] Adding to the positive traits of ALA, scientists are highlighting that ALA also prevents oxidative stress in the aging heart, thus preventing its weakening. Such a nutrition alternative to statin drugs is logical considering its safety, effectiveness, and inexpensive nature.

That heart disease can be prevented or delayed with substances that have anti-inflammatory properties is of paramount importance. The majority (basically the entire world) of medical doctors, natural health practitioners, and purveyors of nutritional supplements are promoting cholesterol lowering via diet, cholesterol lowering drugs, red yeast rice or policosanol. Doing this discounts and often misses the major factor in preventing heart disease: anti-inflammation. Not recognizing such a crucial piece to the heart disease puzzle will inevitably contribute to heart disease.

Let's go ahead and hammer the nail into the cholesterol myth coffin. If it is true that the risk of heart disease rises as blood cholesterol rises, then we should see elevated total cholesterol among those who die early from heart attack. This too has not been the case. Specifically, half of all heart attacks and strokes occur in persons without elevated levels of cholesterol.[122, 123]

---

[121] R.M. Ogborne, S.A. Rushworth, C.A. Charalambos and M.A. O'Connell. "Nrf2 and p38 mediate Alpha Lipoic Acid-Induced Haem Oxygenase-1 Expression in THP-1 Monocytes." *MRC Human Nutrition Research*. Cambridge.

[122] Ridker PM. "Connecting the role of C-reactive protein and statins in cardiovascular disease." *Clinical Cardiology*. 2003 Apr;26(4 Suppl 3): III39-44.

[123] Ridker PM. "Connecting the role of C-reactive protein and statins in cardiovascular disease." *Clinical Cardiology*. 2003 Apr;26(4 Suppl 3): III39-44.

Let's cover the coffin with a layer of cement. If cholesterol caused atherosclerosis, then we would find atherosclerosis throughout the 70,000 miles of arteries within the body through which cholesterol travels. Yet, 90% of the time, atherosclerosis is found in the coronary arteries, while the rest of the arteries remain unharmed by cholesterol.[124] Hence, to say that cholesterol is the culprit is akin to saying that if you jump in water, only your hair will become wet while the rest of your body remains dry. While this may sound absurd to you, so does the cholesterol myth when you consider scientific evidence.

It is estimated that 2700 people die every day from heart disease. Considering the amount of money that is made from the cholesterol lowering myth, the problem is not going away. Pharmaceutical companies are making billions from the sales of cholesterol lowering drugs. The CEO of Pfizer, makers of the popular cholesterol-lowering drug Lipitor, was compensated 33.9 million dollars last year (not including his tens of millions in stock options). This equates to 2.8 million per month, which is about $94,000 per day.

Those who, after reading the evidence, still adhere to the antiquated medical model of lowering cholesterol to prevent heart disease will most likely suffer from it. Adding to this, they may also suffer from the dangers of low cholesterol and thereby decrease their life span.

---

[124] Rath, Matthias, M.D. *Why Animals Don't Get Heart Attacks...But People Do!* Copyright 2003. MR Publishing. ISBN# 0-9679456-8-1.

Myth #7 Cholesterol is Bad for You.

Fact: Cholesterol is vital for most bodily functions. In fact, high cholesterol increases longevity.

Through mass marketing, the pharmaceutical industry has successfully convinced America, and almost the entire world, that cholesterol is bad for you. Succumbing to this, the American Heart Association (AHA), supporting the National Cholesterol Education Program (NCEP) guidelines, has slowly but surely turned every American into a potential patient by asserting that total cholesterol levels should remain below 200 mg/dL in order to prevent heart disease. Fortunately for the pharmaceutical companies, over 105 million Americans have total cholesterol of 200 mg/dL or higher, thereby making millions of people a direct target for their cholesterol lowering drugs.

With the diversity of the human body, as vast as all of the oceans on the planet, how is it that EVERYONE should have the same cholesterol level? Perhaps ALL women should have big breasts and men large penises, right? Or maybe we should all have the exact same heart rate and breathing rate too?

Rather than blindly succumb to rent-a-quote doctors who perpetuate that everyone's cholesterol levels should be below 200 mg/dL, it is vital that everyone obtain a basic understanding of cholesterol and the progression or cause of heart disease. Eventually, you or a loved one will be forced to make vital decisions surrounding some aspect of this issue. This may include making decisions surrounding the use of cholesterol lowering drugs, natural medicine, exercise techniques and/or surgery. Considering that 800 individuals die every day from heart disease, being informed in these matters will be an asset to your health and perhaps even save your life.

Cholesterol has been portrayed by the media and health care industry as akin to poison. This erroneous thinking is the result of billion-dollar marketing campaigns and "selective citation" of cholesterol lowering drug trials. Your understanding of erroneous marketing and selective citation will increase after reading the next few pages.

Cholesterol is a versatile compound that is vital to the function of the human body and just like everything else; cholesterol levels differ greatly among individuals.

In humans, cholesterol serves 5 main functions:

1. Cholesterol is used by the body to manufacture steroids, or cortisone-like hormones, including the sex hormones. These hormones include testosterone, estrogen and cortisone. Combined, these hormones control a myriad of bodily functions.

2. Cholesterol helps the liver produce bile acids. These acids are essential for proper digestion of fats and in ridding the body of waste products.

3. Cholesterol acts to interlock "lipid molecules", which stabilize cell membranes. As such, cholesterol is the building block for all bodily tissues.

4. Most notably, cholesterol is an essential part of the myelin sheath.[125] The myelin sheath, similar to the coating on copper wire, ensures that the brain functions properly by aiding with the passage of electrical impulses. Without the myelin sheath, it is difficult to focus and we can lose memory.

5. And finally, cholesterol has beneficial effects on the immune system. Men with high cholesterol have stronger immune systems than those with low cholesterol, as can be seen by the fact that they have more lymphocytes, total T cells, helper T-cells and CD8+ cells. Further, many strains of bacteria, which cause us to get sick, are almost totally inactivated by LDL cholesterol.[126]

Due to its importance, cholesterol must be circulated to all parts of the body. Therefore, cholesterol circulation is based on the fact that oil and water do not mix. Cholesterol is an oily substance, termed a lipid, and cannot blend smoothly with blood, which is water based. In order to transport this non-water soluble lipid through the bloodstream, the body packages it into special "vehicles" called lipoproteins.

The main cholesterol-carrying vehicle in the body is termed low-density lipoprotein or LDL. Because this LDL carries the lipid known as cholesterol, it is referred to as LDL-

---

[125] Simons M., Kramer E.M., Thiele, C., Stoffel, W., Trotter, J. *Journal of Cellular Biology.* 2000 Oct 2;151(1):143-54.
Bjorkhem I. et al. "Brain Cholesterol: Long Secret Life Behind a Barrier." *Arteriosclerosis, Thrombosis and Vascular Biology.* 2004 Feb 5.

[126] Ravnskov, Uffe. *Quarterly Journal of Medicine* 2003; 96:927-934.

cholesterol. Another form of lipoprotein, and there are numerous forms, is known as high-density lipoprotein, or HDL cholesterol.

The notion that one is bad and the other is good is simply based on the fact that LDL-cholesterol has been found to be one of many components of arterial plaque. Whether it is high or low, LDL cholesterol will still form plaque and damage arteries. Plaque is Nature's "Band Aid" to the damaged inner layer of the artery, known medically as the endothelium. Knowing this and the importance of cholesterol, preventing damage to the endothelium of the arteries sets a precedent over lowering LDL cholesterol levels. To quickly digress, this can be done by ingesting proper amounts of folic acid and B12 to lower a chemical known as homocysteine, which has been shown to damage the endothelial layer of arteries.

Having grasped what cholesterol really is, we can now move on to understanding its relation to heart disease. While complex, it is not hard to learn the basics of how heart disease, or rather atherosclerosis, develops.

Atherosclerosis is an inflammatory response initiated by damage to the innermost layer (known as the endothelium) of the arteries, which faces the bloodstream. This can happen anywhere, but 90% of the time it happens in the arteries of the heart (coronary arteries), probably due to the mechanical stress in this region. Damage to the inner layer of the coronary artery can be attributed to any number of biological disturbances and working to prevent these disturbances is working to prevent atherosclerosis.

Here are a select few:

- Free radical damage leading to oxidized Low Density Lipoproteins (LDL)

- Infection

- Smoking

- High blood pressure

- High blood sugar[127]

- Increased levels of insulin

- Increased levels of homocysteine

- Increased levels of cortisol (i.e. stress)

- Lack of vitamin C

Once damage occurs to the inner layer of the coronary artery, the body's natural repair mechanism takes over. The natural repair mechanism begins with circulating levels of low-density lipoproteins (LDL's) into the damaged area, particularly between the smooth muscle layer and endothelium of the artery.

Once LDL's move into the damaged area of the endothelium, there is an alteration in endothelium function. This alteration begins the inflammation cascade. Most notably, to signal for help, the endothelium begins to produce reactive oxygen species (ROS). This attracts the immune cells to the damaged site. This, in turn, produces growth factors, which cause muscle cells to multiply and invade the damaged area of the blood vessel. Eventually, the conundrum of LDL, immune cells, muscle cells and debris from the initial damage form "plaque."

---

[127] Specifically, high blood sugar leads to advanced glycosylation end products (AGEs), which are compounds found in the blood of diabetics due to an oxidation reaction with excess glucose found in the bloodstream. These scar arterial walls.

Here is the most important thing to understand, plaque is Nature's "Band Aid" for damage to the arterial wall. This "Band Aid" forms whether an individual has high or low LDL. This, in part, explains why researchers have failed to find a correlation between levels of cholesterol and the growth of atherosclerosis.

If damage to the endothelium persists, atherosclerotic plaque accumulates on the arterial walls. This leads to decreased blood flow from the heart, which causes lack of oxygen and nutrients throughout the body. A lack of oxygen and nutrients leads to major problems, involving not only your heart, but also your brain, lungs, kidneys, penile reaction and eventually every body system. Therefore, nutritional supplements that increase blood flow, such as pine bark or grape seed extract, would provide benefit to those who suffer form atherosclerosis by enhancing the delivery of oxygen and nutrients to various parts of the body.

Over time, build up of atherosclerotic plaque initiates heart attack and stroke, sometimes without warning. As an added danger to having plaque buildup, as the artery narrows, tiny blood clots, which are normally harmless, become a death threat. These tiny blood clots, usually capable of passing through a healthy artery, become caught in the plaque and further block the blood flow. If an artery is blocked in the heart, a heart attack is the result. And if a blockage occurs in the brain, a stroke is the result.

To highlight some of the main points of heart disease progression, the body uses numerous substances to form plaque on the arterial walls. This plaque acts as nature's "Band Aid" to heal the inner layer of the arteries. The plaque consists of LDL, immune cells and muscle cells, among other things.

Recognizing that LDL is one of many substances found in plaque and that it carries cholesterol, pharmaceutical companies and medical doctors coined the phrase "bad cholesterol" when referring to LDL. In a weak attempt to support this, they state that LDL is the culprit of deadly plaque buildup. Meanwhile, they ignore the importance of preventing scarring of the mechanically stressed arterial wall, which can be done by lowering homocysteine levels with the proper ratio of folic acid and vitamin B12. Instead, they hold on to the one-dimensional argument, which insists that LDL cholesterol must be lowered to prevent heart disease. In the same breath they prescribe cholesterol-lowering drugs.

Ignoring that the physician should "do no harm," this advice is downright dangerous. Lowering cholesterol has proven life threatening and deadly, especially among the elderly.[128] Hence, if we ignore the evidence, which refutes the cholesterol lowering myth, then it is quite possible that our health will worsen simply due to the dangers associated with having low cholesterol. Repeat that sentence.

Researchers at the University of San Diego highlight that epidemiological studies show that high cholesterol in those over 75 years of age is protective rather than harmful. They state that low cholesterol is a risk factor for heart arrhythmias, which are the leading cause of death if heart attack occurs. Moreover, increased heart arrhythmia (known as atrial fibrillation) due to low cholesterol is an important risk factor for stroke. These researchers conclude that lowering cholesterol does not offer any benefit that exceeds the risk.

Professor Beatriz Rodriquez of the University of Hawaii has also found that low cholesterol among the elderly is not healthy. Reported by BBC News, Professor Beatriz Rodriquez and colleagues found that men over the age of 70 who had cholesterol levels between 200 to 219 milligrams per deciliter

---

[128] Ravnskov, Uffe. *Quarterly Journal of Medicine.* 2003; 96:927-934.

(mg/dL) were less likely to develop heart disease than those with low levels. Elderly men with cholesterol levels of below 160 mg/dL had a 55% greater risk of heart disease.[129]

Other researchers have come to similar conclusions. The *European Heart Journal* has published the results of a 3-year study involving 11,500 patients. Researcher Behar and associates found that in the low cholesterol group (total cholesterol below 160 mg/dL) the relative risk of death was 2.27 times higher compared to those with higher cholesterol. The most common cause of death in the low cholesterol group was cancer, with liver disease being second. The risk of cardiac death was the same in both groups. [130] In support of their findings, these researchers point out that previous studies performed by scientist Keys and associates also showed a higher increase in cancer, particularly lung cancer, when total cholesterol levels were maintained below 170 mg/dL.[131]

More scientists have focused on the link between low cholesterol and cancer. Behar and associates have linked blood cholesterol levels less than 160 mg/dL to a twofold-increased risk of death from cancer of the liver, pancreas and haematopoeitic system. These same researchers also brought to our attention that healthy men, without any history of cardiovascular, gastrointestinal or liver disease, who lower their total cholesterol, have an increased risk of prostate cancer. Also shown is that those with low cholesterol have an increased

[129] BBC News Sunday March 4, 2001. *Low cholesterol "not healthy for elderly"*.

[130] Behar, S. et al. "Low total cholesterol is associated with high total mortality in patients with coronary heart disease." *European Heart Journal.* (1997) 18, 52-59.

[131] Keys. A. Et al. "Serum cholesterol and cancer mortality in seven countries studies." *American Journal of Epidemiology.* 1985:121:870-83.

incidence of death from intracranial hemorrhage, respiratory, kidney and digestive disease.[132]

Looking deeper into the dangers of low cholesterol, it appears that cancer is not the only possible outcome. The chances of early death increase as total cholesterol drops. The most widely respected medical journal, *The Journal of the American Medical Association*, published a study entitled: "Cholesterol and Mortality. 30 Years of Follow-up from the Framingham study." Shocking to most, this in-depth study showed that after the age of 50, there is no increased overall death rate associated with high cholesterol! There was, however, a direct association between low levels (or dropping levels) of cholesterol and increased death. Specifically, medical researchers reported that CVD death rates increased by 14% for every 1 mg/dL drop in total cholesterol levels per year.[133] For example, an individual whose total cholesterol levels dropped 14 mg/dL during 14 years would be expected to have and 11% higher death rate than persons whose cholesterol levels remained constant or rose during the same period.

For those who have already suffered from heart failure, lowering cholesterol may just add to the problem and increase recovery time. The *Journal of Cardiac Failure* published the findings of Horwich and colleagues in a paper entitled "Low Serum Total Cholesterol is Associated with Marked Increase in Mortality in Advanced Heart Failure." In their analysis of 1,134 patients with heart disease, they found that low cholesterol was associated with worse outcomes in heart failure pa-

[132] Behar, S. et al. "Low total cholesterol is associated with high total mortality in patients with coronary heart disease." *European Heart Journal.* (1997) 18, 52-59.

[133] Anderson KM. et al. "Cholesterol and Mortality. 30 Years of Follow-up from the Framingham Study." *Journal of the American Medical Association.* 1987 Apr 24;257(16):2176-80.

tients and impaired survival while high cholesterol improved survival rates. Interesting to note, their findings showed that elevated cholesterol among patients was not associated with hypertension, diabetes, or coronary heart disease.[134]

Low cholesterol has also been linked to depression and anxiety. Duke psychologist Edward Suarez found that women with low cholesterol levels, below 160 mg/dL, were more likely to show signs of depression and anxiety relative to women with normal or high cholesterol levels. In 2003, Duke University showed a 20% absolute increase in depression among those taking cholesterol lowering drugs known as statins. Their results add to the literature linking cholesterol and mood.[135]

The death rate from heart disease has not changed over the last 75 years and mortality from heart failure is more than double what it was in 1996. Thus, those who think they are safe from heart disease due to lowering total cholesterol levels may want to seriously rethink their preventative efforts. Lowering cholesterol, whether by prescription drugs or dietary supplements, would prove dangerous and goes against centuries of scientific research findings, which clearly shows that high cholesterol is protective rather than detrimental.

Combined, these facts are a deathblow to the cholesterol lowering myth and anyone who thinks cholesterol is deadly. As such, they render America's best selling cholesterol lowering drugs useless and in some cases, deadly. Therefore, these facts are among the pharmaceutical industry's biggest secrets.

---

[134] Horwich, et al. "Low serum total cholesterol is associated with marked increase in mortality in advanced heart failure." *Journal of Cardiac Failure.* 2002 Aug;8(4):216-24.

[135] Steffens DC, McQuoid DR, Krishnan KR. "Cholesterol-lowering medication and relapse of depression." *Psychopharmacology Bulletin.* 2003;37(4):92-8.

You won't hear about them from your doctor, the media, or a pharmaceutical sales rep.

This begs the question: How does one successfully convince the entire United States that each and every person should have the same cholesterol level? If this is a myth, then why is it so popular? The belief that low cholesterol prevents heart disease appears to be the result of selective citation rather than scientific results.

Pharmaceutical companies work tirelessly to promulgate the cholesterol-lowering myth by conveniently citing supportive studies while burying the unsupportive. This is known as "selective citation." Reported in the *British Medical Journal* (BMJ), Uffe Ravnskov MD, PhD, shows his results of a meta-analysis of 22 published, controlled, cholesterol-lowering trials. He found that studies considered to be supportive of low cholesterol (typically due to bias) were cited six times more often than those that were unsupportive and that unsupportive trials had not been reported since 1970! Specifically, 8 supportive cholesterol-lowering trials published among major medical journals were cited on average 61 times per year, compared to the 10 unsupportive, which were cited a paltry 8 times per year. Most notably, in 16 trial reports published since 1970, a total of 40 supportive trials were cited while not even a single unsupportive trial was cited. Yet, the number of unsupported trials almost equaled the number of supported. This means that any medical doctor under the age of 35 has never been exposed, via current medical journals, to evidence that refutes the cholesterol lowering myth.[136] Most strikingly, the trials that were often used as "supportive" were false due to the fact that overall death from coronary heart disease was

[136] Ravnskov, Uffe. "Cholesterol lowering trials in coronary heart disease: frequency of citation and outcome." *British Medical Journal.* Volume 305. 4 July 1992.

still unchanged in the trials. So you have perceived benefits that are cited more often, yet the perceived benefits failed to prevent overall death from heart disease.

Preferential citation has skewed the facts by burying the studies that show the importance of cholesterol and its lack of involvement in heart disease. As a result, professionals will continue to teach us that cholesterol is dangerous. And pharmaceutical companies will aggressively push their cholesterol lowering drugs.

In addition to smothering unsupportive studies from our medical history, pharmaceutical companies who sell cholesterol lowering drugs produce brochures, web pages and various other publications to broadcast the cholesterol lowering myth to millions.

As pointed out by the previous editor of the *New England Journal of Medicine*, Jerome P. Kassirer, MD, major publications such as *Lipid Letter*, *Lipids Online*, and *Lipid Management* are supported and funded by cholesterol lowering drug makers. Reaching millions of medical doctors, these publications relentlessly promote the false dangers of cholesterol in an attempt to nudge doctors into prescribing their cholesterol lowering drugs. This ensures not only profit for these drug companies but also promotion of the cholesterol lowering myth.

Hence, preferential citation, combined with paid publications aimed toward medical doctors, guarantees that the pharmaceutical industry can "invent disease" while at the same time provide the remedy. It also guarantees that those who are not privy to the truth behind the cholesterol lowering myth increase their odds of becoming victims to the dangers of low cholesterol.

Myth #8 – Cholesterol Lowering Drugs, known as Statins, are Safe and Effective at Preventing Heart Disease.

Fact: Statins are not effective and any benefits from them are negated by the myriad of negative side effects associated with their use.

According to the AHA, over 105 million Americans have total cholesterol levels of 200 mg/dL or higher. Having convinced the majority of America that cholesterol is dangerous and that total cholesterol levels should be below 200 mg/dL, drug companies have provided a solution for the millions of people who suffer from the perceived problem of high cholesterol: the cholesterol lowering drugs known as "statins."

Commercially, statins are known as atorvastatin (Lipitor), fluvastatin (Lescol), lovastatin (Mevacor), pravastatin (Pravachol), simvastatin (Zocor), and rosuvastatin (Crestor). These drugs were the most widely sold pharmaceutical drugs in 2002. Accounting for 6.5% of the total market share, cholesterol-lowering drugs raked in 12.5 billion dollars! Consequently, you rarely hear the truth surrounding these drugs.

Shane Ellison M.Sc.

Treading on the lunatic fringe, marketing campaigns work aggressively to sell these drugs to every man, women and child under the sun. They do this by asserting that statin drugs are safe and effective for preventing early death from heart disease as well as curing world hunger. Ok, so the last part was an exaggeration, but drug companies are working like mad to convince you that statin drugs are good for treating a barrage of other illnesses, such as Alzheimer's, stiff joints and cancer. And because this is as absurd as curing world hunger, then they may as well tout their statin drugs for that too!

In defense of the safety and effectiveness of statin drugs, drug companies and medical doctors often cite studies known as the "statin drug trials." There have been a myriad of these trials. Most notable are the trials known by their acronyms as ALLHAT, ASCOT-LLA, AFCAPS, WOSCOP, LIPS, GREASE, 4s, HPS, and PROSPER, just to name a few.

These studies were well funded and utilized large populations to analyze the effects of statin drugs on lowering cholesterol and preventing heart disease. Repetitive, mass coverage of the "statin drug trials" has convinced some of the most well-respected health practitioners, medical doctors, and herbalists in the world that lowering cholesterol prevents heart disease. For instance, the wildly marketed book, *The South Beach Diet*, authored by Dr. Agatston, supports the use of statins for lowering cholesterol. The American Heart Association, self-proclaimed authority of cardiovascular health, also promotes the use of cholesterol-lowering drugs. And finally, your family doctor probably adheres to this cholesterol-lowering protocol as well.

At second glance, it is neither logical nor is it scientifically sound to use statin drug trials in defense of lowering cholesterol to prevent heart disease. This is due to the simple fact that statin drug trials have suffered from age and gender bias for close to 10 years. Because all statin drug trials from 1990 to 1999 suffered from both age and gender bias, they eliminated most of the population in their studies, thereby leaving behind valuable information regarding the use of these drugs on other populations. Specifically, statin drug trials were mainly conducted in middle-aged men, and did not study the effects among women, children, and the elderly or ethnic groups.[137] Among these studies were 4S, CARE, LIPID, EXCEL, RE-GRESS, PREDICT, ACAPS, AFCAPS, WOSCOP, KAPS. There were 19 studies in total.

The General Accounting Office of the United States Government has recognized the bias in the statin drug trials as well and stated:

> "The trials generally have not evaluated the efficacy of cholesterol-lowering treatment for several important population groups, such as women, elderly men and women, and minority men and women. Thus, they provide little or no evidence of benefits or possible risks for these groups."

Stressing this point, In 1995, the *Journal of the American Medical Association* (JAMA) also noted that many of the statin drug trials have not included enough women to allow for sex-specific analysis on the effects of statins in women. Researchers Walsh and Grady from the University of California San Francisco highlighted that there is no evidence from primary prevention trials showing that cholesterol-lowering effects among women from the use of statin drugs decreases mortality from heart disease.[138]

---

[137] Bandyopadhyay, S. et al. "Age and Gender in Statin Trials." Quarterly Journal of Medicine. 2001: 94:127-132.

[138] Walsh, J.M., Grady, D. "Treatment of hyperlipidemia in women." *Journal of the American Medical Association.* 1995 Oct 11; 274(14):1152-8.

Shane Ellison M.Sc.

Reiterating this point again in 2004, *JAMA* published results found by researchers at the University of California San Francisco, who reasserted the fact that many of the statin drug trials failed to include enough women in their analyses. To remedy this and to find out whether or not statins are safe and effective for women, researchers combined the results of 13 studies where the impact of statin drugs on women was reported. They found that in women who did not have cardiovascular disease, statin drug use failed to reduce total mortality.[139] Interpreting these results to the masses, reporter Roni Rabin for Newsday.com aptly stated, "We've been bamboozled about cholesterol risks."

That statin drug trials failed to look at the effects of these drugs among the elderly resurfaced in 2004. Recognizing the lack of proof that cholesterol-lowering drugs are safe and affective for the elderly, researchers Holme and colleagues further dissected previous results from statin drug trials. In order to distinguish whether statin drugs are effective or not for the elderly, the statisticians and clinicians reviewed the effects of Pravastatin on the elderly by looking at the statin drug trial known as PROSPER. Adding to the PROSPER findings, they gathered results from other trials where small groups of elderly were used, such as the Heart Protection Study (HPS). Conclusively, these researchers determined that that they found no data to show that statin drugs reduce mortality among the elderly.

Because of this flaw in scientific methodology, one cannot conceivably use the statin drug trials to rationalize prescribing them to the elderly, women of all ages, children or ethnic groups. In other words, prescribing statin drugs to elderly,

---

[139] Walsh, J.M. Pignone, M. "Drug Treatment of hyperlipidemia in women." *Journal of the American Medical Association.* 2004 May 12;291(18):2243-52.

women of all ages and children, as well as those who are not Caucasian, is a giant leap of faith, as safety and effectiveness has not been shown in these populations. If you are among any one of these populations, then you are using a drug that has no studies showing it to be safe and effective. Essentially, you are acting as guinea pig, in the same way users of the previously removed statin drug known as Baycol were. After killing 200 people, Baycol was withdrawn form the market.

Still though, family doctors and medical associations are recommending statin drugs across the board without thinking twice. Whether it is young men, old men, women, blacks, Mexicans and even children, medical doctors are handing out prescriptions for statin drugs. Drug companies are laughing all the way to the bank, as they make billions every year from the false belief that statin drugs are safe and effective for everyone... even your dog Fido.

At the 12th International Symposium on Atherosclerosis, June 2000, Stockholm, Sweden, Dr. Antonio M. Gotto, Jr., dean and medical provost of Cornell University Medical College, predicted that 50% of the entire US population could be taking statin medication. Dr. Antonio M. Gotto told a press conference that he favored this class of drugs for all men aged more than 45 and women aged 55 plus who had a total cholesterol level over 200 mg/dL, an HDL cholesterol of less than 50 mg/dL and one other risk factor for coronary heart disease. This is absolutely baseless and serves as a poignant example of how medical doctors are deceived.

Thinking that the lies and exorbitant use of cholesterol lowering drugs could not get any worse, professionals are unknowingly calling cholesterol-lowering drugs the "new aspirin." More frightening, medical professionals of WebMD are even recommending that children be prescribed cholesterol-

Shane Ellison M.Sc.

lowering drugs![140] Statins are far from being the next aspirin and closer to being the pharmaceutical industry's next "problem child."

Naturally, we can look at the benefits of statins among the population studied in the trials: middle-aged men. Before we do this, we must first understand the definitions of Absolute Risk Reduction vs. Relative Risk Reduction and total mortality. Being alert to this difference is the number one weapon for defending against medical doctors who assume you will blindly take a cholesterol-lowering drug.

Total mortality is the most logical focal point in determining whether or not statin drugs prevent heart disease. Let's elaborate, if one wants to utilize a drug to prevent early death from a given illness, then studies on the particular drug should have results showing that it does in fact prevent early death from the targeted disease while at the same time not eliciting death from all other causes (total mortality). The benefit of using total mortality is two-fold. First, it helps to decipher whether or not the drug works for the prescribed indication. Second, it also helps to determine whether or not the drug caused any deaths from other diseases (i.e. negative side effects). In other words, using the total mortality rate as a focal point of effectiveness ensures that while a drug might prevent a given disease, it does not kill you from cancer, heart attack, or both, hence the term "all-cause."

When reporting total mortality, "absolute" total mortality must be used rather than "relative" total mortality. Don't let medical doctors, drug representatives and "statistical contortionists" convince you otherwise.

---

[140] http://my.webmd.com/content/article/91/100939.htm.

The difference between absolute and relative total mortality rates is a very important distinction. Relative risk reduction (RRR) refers to the percentage decrease in risk achieved by the group receiving the drug. Absolute risk reduction (ARR) refers to the actual difference in risk between the treated and the control group.

Let's look at an example of absolute vs. relative. If drug XYZ prevented the illness known as greed by 10% then the relative risk reduction in greed was 10%. Similarly, looking at the control group, who may have received a "placebo" or sugar pill, they had a 9% relative risk reduction in greed. Therefore, the ABSOLUTE RISK REDUCTION of greed by drug XYZ was 1%. If drug XYZ were to be marketed by the manufacturer, it would be deceitfully advertised that drug XYZ prevents greed by 10%, though in reality it only prevented it by an insignificant 1% (if the manufacturer of drug XYZ paid for the study, then it is likely that the 1% was due to bias).

That the ABSOLUTE RISK REDUCTION was only 1% would be left out of marketing campaigns by the manufacturer of drug XYZ. Instead, they would report to their targeted audience (if it were not a conflict of interest it would most likely be corporate drug pushers) that drug XYZ prevented greed by 10%.

Almost all reports in the popular media and many in medical literature follow this deceitful practice. They present risk results as relative risk reductions rather than absolute risk reductions. This is done to sell more drugs to unsuspecting victims. Relative risk reductions make data seem more impressive than it actually is, especially when it comes to the statin drugs.

When "Absolute Risk Reductions" of total mortality are used as an indicator of the effectiveness of statin drugs, rather than "relative risks" (which are used by the media and doctors

Shane Ellison M.Sc.

to hype drugs and promote their use), statin drug trials fail to show that these drugs prevent early death from total mortality. To quickly highlight this point, we can look to the latest and greatest statin drug Crestor. Crestor plummeted cholesterol levels, yet failed to show any effectiveness as could be seen by a 0% decrease in total mortality rates among users. Thus, the only thing statin drug trials proved was that statin drugs lower cholesterol by inhibiting an enzyme known as HMG-CoA-Reductase. Regardless of their ability to lower cholesterol, they failed to show that this effect has any benefit to preventing early death from heart disease.

Other drugs, such a Pravachol and their respective drug trials show these same tendencies: that there is no correlation between cholesterol levels and prevention of heart disease. This becomes abundantly clear when we look at absolute total mortality rates.

As taught by Joel Kauffman, PhD, Professor of Chemistry Emeritus, the WOSCOPS trial showed only a 0.9% absolute drop in total mortality among those taking the statin drug Pravachol (pravastatin) over 5 years. With respect to heart attack and stroke, the PROSPER trial showed that Pravachol provided no reduction in events among those who had no previous signs of cardiovascular disease (termed primary prevention) and an absolute reduction of 4.3% among those who did (termed secondary prevention).[141] The 4.3% reduction in events was negated by an increase in the incidence of cancer and stroke. Taking a second glance at the rate of cancer among users of Pravachol, we can look to the CARE trial. Accord-

---

[141] Therapeutic Initiative. "Evidence Based Drug Therapy. Do Statins Have a Role in Primary Prevention?" *Therapeutics Letter*. April-May-June 2003. www.ti.ubc.ca.
Therapeutic Initiative. "Evidence Based Drug Therapy. Statins benefit for secondary prevention confirmed." *Therapeutics Letter*. July-September 2003.

ingly, it showed a 1500% increase in cancer among users of Pravachol.

Even the most favorable statin drug trials, having minimal conflicts of interest and ethically sound reporting, the Heart Protection Study (HPS), yielded users of Zocor (simvastatin) with only a 1.8% absolute drop in total mortality. Another trial, the 4S trial, showed a minimal 4% absolute risk reduction in total mortality for those taking Zocor (simvastatin).

The ASCOTT-LLA trial, designed to identify the benefits of Lipitor, (atorvastatin) showed 0% reduction in absolute total mortality rates among those taking Lipitor. Looking at absolute reduction of heart attack and stroke, Lipitor (atorvastatin) yielded a miniscule reduction of 1.2% over 3.3 years.[142]

Researchers from *Therapeutic Initiatives* performed a meta-analysis[143] of 5 major statin drug trials, these being PROSPER, ALLHAT-LLT, ASCOT-LLA, AFCAPS and WOSCOPS. In the pooled data of these trials, statin drugs provided a total Absolute Risk Reduction in total mortality of 0.3% among those who showed no signs of having cardiovascular disease (primary prevention).[144] With respect to preventing heart attack and stroke, the five combined studies showed that statins

---

[142] Kauffman, JM. "Bias in Recent Papers on Diets and Drugs in Peer-Reviewed Medical Journals." *Journal of the American Physicians and Surgeons.* 2004;9(1).

[143] A meta-analysis is a statistical procedure to combine a number of existing studies. Through such a procedure, effects that are hard or impossible to discern in the original studies because of a too-small sample size can be made visible, as the meta-analysis is (in the ideal case) equivalent to a single study with the combined size of all original studies. A weakness of the method is that problems with any of the studies will affect the result of the meta-analysis, so a good meta-analysis of bad studies will still result in bad data.

[144] Therapeutics Initiative. "Evidence Based Drug Therapy. Do Statins have a Role in Primary Prevention?" April-May-June 2003. The University of British Columbia. www.ti.ubc.ca.

prevented these events by a mere 1.4%. Utilizing LIPS, PROSPER, GREASE, and HPS, a meta-analysis shows that statin use prevented total mortality by 1.8% among those who showed signs of having cardiovascular disease (secondary prevention).[145]

The statin drug trials make it clear that the drugs lower cholesterol while providing little to no benefit of heart disease prevention. Utilizing L-arginine, pine bark, vitamin C, a combo of B12 and folic acid, and/or omega-3 fatty acids would provide significantly greater protection from heart disease (see end of chapter for details). Relative to statin drugs, the use of these nutrients would not be accompanied with negative side effects and inflated costs.

As the incidence of heart disease continues to grow, so will the availability of prescription drugs that are purported to prevent or heal. Most recently, the "polypill" serves as a perfect example. As the love affair with profits from statin drugs continues, so-called experts are now recommending that they be combined with other drugs.

Hailed as a "strategy to reduce cardiovascular disease by more than 80%," authors and patent holders to the concoction assert that everyone should use this pill over the age of 55.[146] Yes, everyone on the entire planet. Can you believe that daring assertion by so-called scientists?

---

[145] Therapeutics Initiative. "Evidence Based Drug Therapy. Statins Benefit for Secondary Prevention Confirmed. What is the optimal dosing strategy?" *Therapeutics Letter.* July-September 2003. The University of British Columbia. www.ti.ubc.ca.

[146] Wald, N.J. Law, M. R. "A strategy to reduce cardiovascular disease by more than 80%." *British Medical Journal.* 2003. June 28; 326 (7404):1419.

Wald and Law propose a cocktail of a statin drug, three blood pressure lowering drugs, an angiotensin-converting enzyme inhibitor, folic acid and aspirin to be used to battle heart disease. That these "scientists" would recommend such heavy use of drugs is laughable and sad all at the same time.

Their assertion is based on an analysis done by computer, which looked at all previous studies of the individual components of the drug stack. In other words, they failed to do any medical examination whatsoever. They never studied the interactions that these drugs might have with each other once consumed as the 'polypill'. They never studied the long-term effects of the 'polypill'. And they never considered whether or not it is safe among men, women, the elderly or ethnic groups! Not to mention that the main ingredient, a statin drug, is among the most dangerous drugs ever promoted for human consumption. Yet, these patent holders can get away with making false claims for an imaginary drug and recommend its use among EVERYONE over the age of 55, all based on computer evaluation. This is incredulous. Trailblazers of the scientific method are rolling over in their graves.

The only thing that could disgrace the scientific community more would be the approval of leading journal editors. And not surprisingly, this is exactly what happened. The editor of the *British Medical Journal* (*BMJ*) appears to have sold his soul to pharmaceutical interests. Upon release of the biased paper, his suggestion was that we "keep this issue of the *BMJ*. It may well become a collector's item. It's perhaps more than 50 years since we published something as important as the cluster of papers from Nick Wald, Malcolm Law, and others." He is right on one point. This paper published by the *BMJ* is a collector's edition. Never in the history of the *BMJ* have they ever published such absurdity. Never in the history of the *BMJ* have they recommended a pill to an entire population without any one ever studying its real-life effects or even swallowing the damn thing! Never!

Statins are a textbook case of the "cure" being more deadly than the disease, and this is when they are used alone. To combine them with other drugs would be a death sentence.

Any benefits from statin drugs are canceled by negative side effects. These dangers rarely discussed. Unknown to the public and most doctors, cholesterol lowering drugs can be life threatening.[147] In a letter to the *Archives of Internal Medicine*, Uffe Ravnskov MD, PhD and colleagues show that in two of the three clinical trials that included healthy people, the chance of survival was better without the use of cholesterol lowering drugs.[148] Numerous medical journals have shown that cholesterol-lowering drugs significantly increase one's risk of suffering from loss of memory (transient global amnesia) and loss of mental focus, cancer, CoQ10 deficiency (paradoxically, low CoQ10 leads to congestive heart failure), rhabdomyolysis, and erectile dysfunction.

Because cholesterol works to ensure the integrity of the myelin sheath (responsible for carrying electrical messages throughout the brain for memory and focus), a logical hypothesis is that lowering it can have a negative effect on memory and focus. Observing the effects of statin drugs, which significantly lower cholesterol, we find that this hypothesis may hold true among users. Dr. Graveline, MD, a NASA astronaut, flight surgeon, family doctor and author of "Lipitor – Thief of Memory," claims he lost his memory after six weeks of using Lipitor. From his testimony we learn that he could not recognize his house or his wife after using the statin drug

---

[147] Cohen, S. Jay. *Over Dose.* 2001. ISBN 1-58542-123-5.
[148] Uffe Ravnskov, et al. "Letter to Archives of Internal Medicine." Submitted on July 20, 2002.

Lipitor. His memory loss lasted for six hours at a time. After quitting the drug, his lapses in memory ceased.

Dr. Graveline is not alone in his experience. Loss of memory from using statin drugs has become so widespread it has caught the attention of CBS News, who reported the findings of researcher Dr. Beatrice Golomb, assistant professor of medicine at the University of California in San Diego. She states that: "We have people who have lost thinking ability so rapidly [from using statins] that within the course of a couple of months they went from being head of major divisions of companies to not being able to balance a checkbook and being fired from their company."[149]

Most notably, it appears that cholesterol-lowering drugs also increase one's risk of developing cancer. In their study published in the *Journal of the American Medical Association* (*JAMA*), Thomas B. Newman, MD, MPH, and co-workers show that all cholesterol lowering drugs, both the early drugs known as fibrates (glofibrate, gemfibrozil) and the newer drugs known as statins (Lipitor, Pravachol, Zocor), cause cancer in rodents at the equivalent doses used by man.[150]

Interestingly, these facts are not reflected in the highly coveted Physicians Desk Reference (PDR). For instance, the PDR shows that cancer is a side effect for fibric acid derivates and statins only when as much as 10 times of the recommended human dose is used. This is a blatant lie.

Dr. Gloria Troendle, deputy director for the Division of Metabolism and Endocrine Drug Products for the FDA, noted

---

[149] O'Fallon, Ill., May 24, 2004. *CBS Evening News.* "Statins' Mind-Boggling Effects."

[150] Newman, Thomas B. et al. "Carcinogenicity of Lipid-Lowering Drugs." *Journal of the American Medical Association.* January 3, 1996-Vol 275, No. 1.

that the cholesterol-lowering drug gemfibrozil belonged to a class of drugs that has repeatedly been shown to increase death rates among users. Moreover, Dr. Troendle stated that she does not believe the FDA has ever approved a drug for long-term use that was as cancer causing at human doses as gemfibrozil.

Others shared these same concerns about gemfibrozil. Elizabeth Barbehenn, PhD, concluded to the FDA, "fibrates must be considered as potential human carcinogens and their carcinogenic potential should be part of the risk benefit equation for evaluating gemfibrozil."

Ignoring these facts, the pharmaceutically campaigned FDA approved these drugs, despite having a majority vote among their advisory committee! Specifically, when asked to vote whether or not the cholesterol-lowering drug gemfibrozil should be approved for prevention of heart disease, only 3 out of 9 voted in favor of approval. Unfortunately, these votes are only "advisory" and the FDA decided to approve gemfibrozil for human consumption against the better judgment of the committee.

Of course, the extrapolation of evidence of cancer from rodent to human is very uncertain. And this is the argument of those in favor of using cholesterol-lowering drugs. The argument would be plausible in that such an extrapolation would only hold true if human studies also showed an increase in cancer rates. And in fact, that is what scientists are seeing. Reported in the *Lancet*, Shepard and colleagues for PROSPER noted that "new cancer diagnoses were more frequent on pravastatin [Pravachol] than on placebo [those not taking the drug]".[151] Evidence from the cholesterol-lowering drug trial known as

---

[151] Shepard, J. et al. "Pravastatin in elderly individuals at risk of vascular disease (PROSPER): a randomized controlled trial." *Lancet*. 2002 Nov 23:360(9346):1623-30.

CARE (Cholesterol And Recurrent Events) showed a 1500% increase in breast cancer among women taking Pravachol (a cholesterol-lowering drug made by Bristol-Myer Squib).[152]

In a huge blow to the statin-dealing drug camp, Dr. Joseph Mercola outlines the mechanism by which cholesterol-lowering drugs cause cancer. As published in *Nature Medicine,* Dr. Michael Simons of Beth Israel Deaconess Medical Center in Boston shows that statin drugs mimic a substance known as vascular endothelial growth factors (VEGF). The biochemical VEGF promotes the growth of new blood vessels, a process known as angiogenesis. While angiogenesis may help the growth of arteries, the benefit is quickly negated by the potential for growth of cancer. Specifically, the *British Journal of Cancer* reports that VEGF plays an important role in the spread of colorectal cancer. Further, for those who already have tumors, VEGF significantly diminishes their survival time.[153, 154]

The fact that cholesterol-lowering drugs can potentially cause cancer at doses commonly used by humans will never be accepted as mainstream knowledge. Drug company-funded studies for cholesterol lowering drugs are conveniently short in nature, typically 5 years or less. It takes decades for cancer to develop. In fact, even heavy smoking will not cause lung cancer within 5 years.[155] Yet it is a well-known fact that smoking leads to lung cancer. Therefore, as long as statin drug trials

[152] *New England Journal of Medicine.* 1996 Oct 3;335(14):1001-9. http://www.ravnskov.nu/ncep_guidelines.

[153] Akagi K. et al. "Vascular endothelial growth factor-C (VEGF-C) expression in human colorectal cancer tissues." *British Journal of Cancer.* 2000 Oct;83 (7):887-91.

[154] *Nature Medicine.* September 2000;6:965-966, 1004-1010.

[155] Ravnskov, Uffe. "Statins as the new aspirin." Letters. *British Medical Journal.* 2002; 324:789 (30 March).

last only 5 years, this side effect will continue to fly below the radar.

The list of negative side effects from cholesterol-lowering drugs goes on. Researchers from the University of Denmark report that about 15% of cholesterol-lowering drug users over the age of 50 will suffer from nerve damage as a direct result of using statin drugs.[156] USA Today reported, "Statins have killed and injured more people than the government has acknowledged."[157]

Learning about the number of negative side effects associated with cholesterol-lowering drugs makes one wonder what the hell is going on! The negative side effects or serious adverse events (SAE) mentioned above are not well known among medical doctors simply because they are rarely published. For instance, the *British Medical Journal* (*BMJ*) has reported that of 164 statin drug trials reviewed; only 48 reported the number of participants with one or more negative side effects caused by the drug.[158] *Therapeutics Letter* reports that among the trials that did report SAE's, they failed to identify what the SAE's were.[159]

Fortunately, 50% of those who take cholesterol-lowering drugs quit within the first year due to negative side effects. Considering that medical doctors utilize the statin drug trials as their primary source of information, it is unlikely that the 50% of patients who stay on cholesterol lowering drugs will ever

[156] Julie Appleby and Steve Sternberg, *USA Today.* 08/20/2002.

[157] Sternberg, Steve. *USA Today.* 08/20/2001.

[158] Law, M.R. et al. "Quantifying effect of statins on low density lipoprotein cholesterol, ischaemic heart disease, and stroke: systematic review and meta-analysis." *British Medical Journal.* 2003, June 28; 326 (7404): 1423.

[159] Wright, M. Jim. et al. "Analysis of serious adverse events. Lipid-lowering therapy revisited." *Therapeutics Letter.* 2001;42:1-3.

become aware of the serious adverse events associated with cholesterol lowering drugs, even when they fall victim to them.

The cost of these drugs explains their popularity. Not able to patent natural medications, drug companies would be out of business overnight if the masses began utilizing these nutrients instead of statin drugs. And considering the money that drug companies pump into research labs, many scientists would be forced out of jobs. To add to the financial crisis that would occur, pharmaceutical stocks would plummet. Thus, it is the financial benefit, not the health benefits, which makes these drugs successful. As a consequence, it is rare that the masses would learn of the benefits of the aforementioned nutrients.

To ensure that you do not fall victim to the hype and greed, here are three questions to ask your doctor before filling the prescription:

- What is the ABSOLUTE reduction in total mortality rates among users of the drug?

- What are the negative side effects of using the drug?

- Are there any natural alternatives?

If these questions cannot be answered to your satisfaction, think twice before filling the prescription. Statin drugs do not prevent early death from heart disease, despite their cholesterol lowering effects. Greedy drug manufacturers and statistical contortionists who work relentlessly to prove that statin drugs are safe and effective have hoodwinked medical doctors and patients.

Nutrition Cocktails for Complete Risk Reduction of Heart Disease

The risk of suffering from heart disease is determined by numerous factors. Focusing on one factor, while ignoring

Shane Ellison M.Sc.

others, inevitably increases our chances of suffering from this top killer. In contrast, focusing on numerous factors could potentially afford complete risk reduction. Such factors include restoring endothelial function, lowering platelet aggregation (preventing clots), moderating blood pressure, increasing blood circulation, preventing plaque buildup, using an anti-inflammatory, preventing oxidative stress with an antioxidant, providing the heart with optimal energy in the form of fatty acids, lowering homocysteine levels, and preventing insulin resistance. Several nutritional supplements have proven beneficial in the pursuit of complete risk reduction of heart disease.

L-Arginine (2 to 6 grams daily) and Pine Bark (100-200 mg daily)- L-arginine, a nitric oxide (NO) donor, and pine bark work synergistically, meaning that their combined use provides greater benefits than when used individually.

A major factor in the development of atherosclerosis is endothelial dysfunction. Endothelial dysfunction results in loss of dilation, constriction, the obstruction of blood vessels by clots, and inflammation. In total, if a person suffers from endothelial dysfunction, their body is unable to deliver blood, nutrients, and oxygen throughout the body. Additionally, endothelial dysfunction would result in the body's inability to deliver components of the immune system throughout the body. Hypothetically speaking, this would lead to other forms of illness. This might explain chronic illness among the elderly who show signs of heart disease. Endothelial dysfunction also predicts type-2 diabetes in women independent of other known risk factors.[160]

L-Arginine prevents endothelium dysfunction. It also improves endothelium dysfunction for those who already suffer

---

[160] James, B. et al. "Biomarkers of Endothelial Dysfunction and Risk of Type 2 Diabetes Mellitus." *Journal of the American Medical Association.* 2004;291:1978-1986.

from it, as can be seen by its effectiveness among those who have hypertension (a sign of endothelial dysfunction). In addition to improving or ensuring vascular health, L-arginine works to prevent type-2 diabetes as well as improve exercise duration.

Elderly men will be happy to know that L-arginine, when combined with pine bark, does wonders for enhancing penile erection. Relative to the placebo group, absolute restored sexual ability has been shown to be increased by a whopping 75% among users of both L-arginine and pine bark.[161]

Studied extensively at the University of Arizona by Ronald Watson, PhD, pine bark has a myriad of preventative effects for those looking to prevent heart disease. Pine bark consists of chemicals known as procyanidins: polymers of catechin and epicatechin sub units (also found in grape seed extract, perhaps less expensive than pine bark). Most notably, pine bark lowers and prevents platelet aggregation without any negative side effects when used for at least 2 months. Abnormal platelet aggregation increases the risk of blood clots, which in turn increases the risk of heart attacks and strokes. Aspirin is often used for this purpose, though pine bark has shown to be more effective and safer, as it does not increase bleeding times or gastrointestinal bleeding. Pine bark has also been shown to lower high blood pressure (-20%) and to improve circulation (resulting in better delivery of oxygen and nutrients throughout the body). [162]

Vitamin C (2 to 20 grams daily) – Humans are one of the only animals on the planet whose body does not manufacture vitamin C, but need it for survival. Therefore, all humans

[161] Stanislavov, R. et al. "Treatment of erectile dysfunction with pycnogenol and L-arginine." *Journal of Sex and Marital Therapy.* 2003 May-Jun;29(3):207-13.

[162] Watson, Ronald. *Evidence Based Integrative Medicine.* 2003:1(1) 27-32.

need to ingest 2-20 grams of vitamin C daily, throughout their entire life, in order to maintain good health status. That you only need a few hundred milligrams, as advised by the FDA, is laughable. This is like saying you only need a few ounces of water daily, while hiking in the desert.

Vitamin C has many roles. But of paramount importance is its role in preventing the breakdown of the 60,000 miles worth arteries, veins and capillaries that reside in our body. By preventing this breakdown, vitamin C prevents excess plaque buildup. Vitamin C does this by serving as a production factory for collagen and elastin, which serve to strengthen arteries, veins and capillaries. This strengthening prevents the inflammation process of heart disease in its tracks.

Vitamin C also lowers levels of a chemical in our body known as homocysteine. Homocysteine is an amino acid and considered a risk factor for heart disease due to its ability to damage the endothelium (inner layer of the arteries facing the bloodstream). As learned previously, such damage leads to plaque buildup. Therefore, high levels of homocysteine lead to a greater chance of suffering from heart disease. Therefore, rather than being a symptom of heart disease, high levels of homocysteine are a cause. Scientist David Wall and associates, publishing their findings in the *British Medical Journal*, showed that lowering homocysteine levels reduced the risk of heart disease by 16%, the obstruction of blood vessels by clot formation by 25% and stroke by 24%.[163]

Alpha-Lipoic Acid (ALA) (600 mg/day) and Acetyl-L-Carnitine (ALCAR) (2g/day) – ALA and ALCAR are two more vital nutritional supplements that, when used together, provide significant benefits through synergy. As we age, quan-

[163] Wald, David. Et al. "Homocysteine and cardiovascular disease: evidence on causality from meta-analysis." *British Medical Journal.* 2002;325:1202 (23 November).

tities of both ALA and ALCAR begin to decline in the body. Therefore, the Linus Pauling Institute of Oregon State University considers both ALA and ALCAR "age-essential" micronutrients.

ALA acts as an anti-inflammatory to prevent plaque build up. It also serves to prevent the development of insulin resistance and oxidative stress in the aging heart, thus keeping the heart strong as we age. Specifically, as an antioxidant, ALA inhibits the "hydroxyl radical." The hydroxyl radical is considered to be the most damaging of the free radicals due to its ability to initiate "lipoprotein peroxidation." Lipoprotein peroxidation creates the "oxidized LDL molecule." This is of paramount importance in that if the hydroxyl radical is not inhibited, then the "oxidized LDL molecule" might cause undesirable health problems such as atherosclerosis.

ALCAR is a molecular chaperone to essential fatty acids, helping to ensure that they are delivered to the cell's furnace, the mitochondria, to be burned as fuel. Using ALCAR ensures that the heart receives energy in the form of fatty acids, the sole fuel used by this most important muscle. By providing fatty acids to the heart, the heart avoids an energy deficit, thereby further preventing it from weakening.

Lonnis Rizos of the University of Athens Medical School documented a 15% decrease in absolute mortality rates among those patients who suffered from heart failure and supplemented with ALCAR for 3 years.[164] Most striking is that these patients already had a weakening heart from previous heart failure and did not use ALA in conjunction with ALCAR, yet still managed to significantly decrease mortality rates.

Polyphenols (from food source daily) – Polyphenols are found in common foods or nutritional supplements including

---

[164] Rizos Lonnis. *American Heart Journal.* Volume 139, Number 2, Part 3.

Shane Ellison M.Sc.

but not limited to olive oil and green tea. To highlight the effectiveness of polyphenols for preventing heart disease we can look to a single study, The Lyon Diet Heart Study. This study compared a Mediterranean diet (rich in olive oil) to a standard "Westem diet" in patients who had suffered from a heart attack. After 27 months, those who had a diet rich in olive oil showed a 76-percent reduction in cardiac events.[165] Incorporating polyphenol rich foods or tea into a healthy eating plan would prove beneficial. Polyphenols are potent anti-inflammatory agents as well as antioxidants. Their sum effect is the prevention of plaque buildup.

B6 (12.5 mg), B12 (500mcg) and Folic Acid (400 mcg) – Daily administration of these three nutrients (either from diet or supplements) effectively lowers homocysteine levels. Doing so would protect the endothelium from damage and subsequent plaque build up. This stack also provides protection from cancer and depression.

Exericse - Exercise is an excellent way to enhance or restore endothelial dysfunction. Moreover, exercise increases the benefits obtained from nutritional supplements. Scientists at the University of California at Los Angeles (UCLA) show that both exercise and nutritional supplementation provide a "synergistic effect" by protecting the arteries from the inflammation process, which leads to atherosclerosis. Their findings were published by the *Proceedings of the National Acedemy of Sciences*.

---

[165] Patrick, Lynn. "Cardiovascular Disease: C-reactive Protein and the Inflammatory Disease Paradigm: HMG-CoA Reductase Inhibitors, alpha-Tocopherol, Red Yeast Rice, and Olive Oil Polyphenols. A Review of the Literature."

Myth #9 – Ephedra causes Heart Attack, Stroke and Seizures.

Fact: Ephedra has been used safely for thousands of years.

The complex issues surrounding natural medicine makes it downright difficult to understand the benefits and dangers associated with ephedra's use. This is a great asset to the pharmaceutically compliant media. Using this asset, they are able to run a few smear campaigns on CNN and within hours, whip every American into a frenzy concerning the natural medicine at issue. Using this momentum to their advantage, lawmakers are quick to pass bills forbidding the use of natural medicines. This is exactly what happened with Ephedra, its Chinese name being Ma Huang, despite the fact that it is as safe as caffeine.

The FDA and the United States Department of Health and Human Services (HHS) have asserted that ephedra poses an unnecessary risk for suffering from heart attacks, stroke and seizures. This has been regurgitated in every paper in America. And, without thinking twice, the evidence supporting this assertion, or rather, the lack of evidence, was accepted by the general public and medical doctors without hesitation. Thanks to this blind loyalty, ephedra is now thought to Mother Nature's weapon for mass destruction. In truth, you are more likely to be killed from a bee sting than die from consuming ephedra.

Ephedra was among the first plants used for medicinal purposes over an estimated 5000 years ago. It is native to China, but also found in the Mediterranean region, India, Persia, and the western portion of South America. It is known botanically as *Ephedra sinica*.

The active ingredients in ephedra are referred to as alkaloids. The main alkaloid is the molecule known as ephedrine, making up about 1.25-8% of the plant by weight. Other alkaloids found in ephedra include pseudoephedrine, methylephedrine, norephedrine, methylpseudoephedrine and norpseudoephedrine.

Reading the labels of several over-the-counter drugs, you will notice that the same alkaloids in ephedra are also found in many pharmaceutical preparations. These include nose drops, cold tablets, cough syrups and asthma relief medications. Prior to its ban, over 2 billion doses of ephedra were being consumed every year in America. In business terms, this equates to a loss of 2 billion doses that would have otherwise been consumed via these pharmaceutical counterparts. Hence, the turf wars against ephedra.

Paradoxically, the naturally occurring alkaloids ephedrine and norephedrine, marketed under the name phenylpropanolamine, are manufactured by drug companies and are FDA approved drugs. Both can be obtained over the counter at gas stations or from a medical doctor. The FDA considers these forms of the drug safe for consumption by both adults and children, as can be seen by its FDA approval. In contrast, if these alkaloids are consumed by taking ephedra, the FDA asserts that it poses significant risk to health and can even kill you.

Rarely are ephedrine and ephedra differentiated in the media. As a result, ephedra is often blamed for negative results from using the pharmaceutical counterpart, ephedrine. Understanding the distinction between the two enables one to better understand the lazy reporting done by the media and medical doctors.

Ephedra is a plant and contains a myriad of alkaloids in very small proportions. Ephedrine is sold in pill form as ephedrine HCl. Ultimately, ephedra is far safer than ephedrine. It is well documented that the key benefit that ephedra has over the synthetic counterpart ephedrine is that it is slowly released into the bloodstream. Conversely, ephedrine is released at a much faster rate, delivering a large amount of the drug into the bloodstream quickly. This fast absorbing version can often lead to signs of overdose such as rapid heart rate, heavy breathing, sweating and insomnia.

Ephedra, like caffeine, is a stimulant. It activates the sympathetic nervous system. Depending on how much is consumed, activation elicits excitement within the body that would be akin to having a sexual encounter, or initiating the "fight or flight" response within the body. Therefore, logic dictates that if ephedra poses "unreasonable risk," so does having sex or getting overtly excited.

The pharmacology of how ephedra works in the body can be extensive. For the sake of over simplifying, we will look at a few of the main points. The effects of ephedra are mediated by its activation of receptors found throughout the body known as α_1, β_1 and β_2 receptors of the adrenergic system. Once done, this elicits the following actions in the body:

- Activation of lypolysis, the release of fat from fat stores

- Stimulation of thyroid metabolism via alpha-adrenergic mediation

- Bronchodilation, or the opening of bronchial tubes to increase oxygen consumption

- Enhanced energy capacity due to Increased blood flow to the muscles, providing for an increased supply of oxygen and blood-borne nutrients

- Elevation of mood, motivation and concentration

The main problem with ephedra is its short half-life. In an effort to ensure that the action of ephedra is maintained for longer periods, many individuals consume an exorbitant amount. This inevitably results in negative side effects such as dry mouth, angina, nervousness or insomnia. But rarely does anyone die. In fact, The American Association of Poison Control Centers' (AAPCC) annual report documented only 1 death from the wrongful use of the herb ephedra (compare this to the 16,500 NSAID-related deaths occur each year among arthritis patients). These side effects are easily remedied when doses of ephedra are kept within reasonable limits, such as 50-80 mg per day. Like everything else, ephedra must be used properly. Professional sport teams failed to take note of this hypocrisy, and instead of banning NSAIDS, they banned ephedra. This gave more support to the United States government's false claims surrounding ephedra. Way to go NFL.

Ephedra Unplugged

Seriously, are we so brainwashed by television that we believe lawmakers are protecting us when they work to ban natural plants such as ephedra? Of course we are!

Millions of fat Americans sit in front of their boob tube slurping their coffee in the morning as they watch CNN report how deadly ephedra can be. Never mind that in 1999 alone, the federal government's Drug Abuse Warning Network (DAWN) reported 427 deaths involving acetaminophen and 104 involving aspirin.[166]

Meanwhile, Joe Coffee scurries to work; and, like a parrot, tells everyone how "deadly ephedra can be." After all, he is now an expert from the simple act of glazing at the "tube." It's sad, after 35 years of being alive Joe Coffee still cannot take part in the great American pass time called "thinking."

It seems that the fears of ephedra have caused amnesia among Americans, as they have forgotten that it has successfully been used for over 5000 years to treat a myriad of afflictions, most notably obesity, which they suffer from terribly. Additionally, when mixed with other herbs, its safety profile makes coffee appear poisonous.

To further substantiate ephedra's safety, we can look to the US General Accounting Office (GAO). In 1999, the US General Accounting Office (GAO) made a report to congress stating that the Federal Drug Administration (FDA) Adverse Events Reports (AERs) surrounding ephedra (commonly used as an argument against ephedra) were "poorly documented." It appeared that the amount of product used, how often it was used, and for how long it was used was not substantiated. The GAO continued to report that 10 to 73 percent of the so-called AERs were not even associated with ephedra![167]

Believe it, Joe Coffee. The pharmaceutical lap dog known as the FDA lied to you! Feeling depressed about this?

---

[166] Sullum, Jacob. *USA Today*. Mclean, VA. July 1, 2002. Page A11.
[167] "Dietary Supplements. Uncertainties in Analyses Underlying FDA's Proposed Rule on Ephedrine Alkaloids." GAO/HEHS/GGD-99-90.

Perhaps you should try some Prozac. The world needs fewer idiots!

Playing devils advocate, 100 so-called (often announced on the airwaves) deaths attributed to the use of ephedra pales in comparison to the number of deaths caused by tobacco, FDA approved drugs and medical doctors. For instance, cigarettes kill about 400,000 per year, the *Journal of the American Medical Association* reports that medical doctors are the number three killer in the USA and synthetic drugs number four![168]

Let the facts speak for themselves, that ephedra has been responsible for nearly 100 deaths and 1,178 adverse reactions is a fallacy. Of course, ephedra, like sugar, must be used properly and most supplement companies have ignored this. Nonetheless, ephedra is in fact an inexpensive natural product that poses huge competition to pharmaceutical companies. Most notably, ephedra is poised to successfully treat obesity, manage the symptoms of ADHD, depression and asthma, when used correctly.

Considering that obesity kills 800 people per day and that the American Cancer Society has stated that obesity may soon be the leading cause of cancer, it would appear that ephedra is exactly what America needs!

The FDA mounted its first case against ephedra using its Adverse Reaction Monitoring System. It was highly touted by them and various other medical authorities, such as the Mayo Clinic, that from 1995 to 1997 there were 926 cases of possible ephedra toxicity leading to stroke, heart attack and sud-

---

[168] *Journal of the American Chemical Society*. July 26, 2000-Vol 284, No.4.

den death based on the Adverse Event Reports (AER) reported by the Adverse Reaction Monitoring System.[169]

News spread faster than a brush fire on a windy day. Reacting to this report by the FDA, medical doctors quickly authored papers touting the dangers of ephedra based on the so-called AERs. For instance, the *New England Journal of Medicine* reported that based on AERs from the FDA: "The use of dietary supplements that contain ephedra alkaloids may pose a health risk to some persons." Johns Hopkins University insisted that using ephedra would lead to serious side effects such as heart attacks, strokes, arrhythmias, increased blood pressure and heart palpitations. Additionally, they reminded us that ephedra was not FDA approved and that most clinical studies examining ephedra for weight loss have documented adverse effects in 20 percent to 60 percent of patients. They failed to document specifically which studies they were referring to simply because these studies do not exist.

Further, using the ephedra scare to ignite an all-out war on all dietary supplements, the *Journal of the America Medical Association* published the writing of Phil B. Fontanarosa, MD. Dr. Fontanarosa used the false ephedra AERs to assert, "Dietary supplements should be subject to more rigorous regulation by the FDA."[170]

This false reporting was far more dangerous than the ephedra itself.

The reports alone, with their blatant scare tactics, gave almost every user of ephedra an immediate heart attack, or so they thought. Money hungry law offices joined in by offering

---

[169] Samenuk, David. *Mayo Clinic Proceedings.* 2002; 77:12-16.

[170] Fontanarosa, Phil B. *Journal of the American Medical Association.* 2003:289:1568-1570.

to sue any and all companies selling products that contained ephedra. Madness set in and ephedra's reputation was scarred forever thanks to so-called Adverse Event Reports (AERs) from the FDA.

Few reporters and medical doctors failed to learn that the AERs had already been discounted by the US General Accounting Office (GAO) as an unworthy source for determining whether or not ephedra was dangerous. Specifically, authors such as Dr. David Samenuk and Dr. Fontanarosa failed to recognize that AERs from the FDA reflect only reported data and do NOT represent scientific methodology. For instance, AERs provide no patient history, treatment history nor do they give a description of confounding factors that might discount a true relation to ephedra and an AER. In other words, the AERs often fail to show a true correlation between the use of ephedra and negative side effects. As a result, they cannot be relied upon to establish a causal relationship between ephedra use and negative side effects. Doing so goes against thousands of years of learned and accepted scientific methodology. That these authors relied on AERs and published their results in leading scientific journals demonstrates a misunderstanding of scientific methodology, a disgrace to themselves and others in their profession.

Acknowledging that if the Adverse Reaction Monitoring System were accurate, then America would have a public health crisis based on its results, the GAO stepped in. The GAO effectively separated fiction from reality with respect to the AERs.

Most strikingly, the GAO noted that when reviewing the AERs, the FDA instructed medical doctors not to use the standard scientific definition of "adverse events," but instead use their "clinical judgment" in determining whether or not ephedra caused a serious event. This initial analysis, which abandoned the scientific method immediately, discounts AERs related to ephedra and consequently resulted in a myriad of shortcomings in the case against ephedra. These shortcomings were rarely if at all spoken about in the media. They were as follows:

- 39% lacked information on the amount of ephedra consumed. Was it 5 mg or 1000 mg?

- 41% lacked information on the frequency with which ephedra was used. Were they taking it once per day or every hour of the day?

- 28% lacked information on the duration for which the product was used. Had they been using it for 10 minutes or 10 years?

- And finally, the 13 most cited AERs by the FDA to defend the restriction of ephedra involved the pharmaceutical drug ephedrine, not ephedra! Apparently the medical doctors, hired by the FDA, either did not or could not differentiate between the synthetic drug ephedrine and the plant ephedra. Therefore, if any conclusion is to be made from AERs, it would be that the FDA approved drug ephedrine was dangerous, not ephedra.

The GAO concluded that based on scientific evidence and not on clinical judgment, it appears that the use of synthetic ephedrine, not ephedra, can result in adverse experiences. Most importantly, it was noted that the FDA AERs do not provide sufficient evidence on which to base any regulatory rule on ephedra.

The FDA lost its battle against ephedra to science. As a result, ephedra stayed on the market and millions of people continued to use it. Their benefits being continued fat loss and the choice to use either the pharmaceutical concoctions or the natural plant. Meanwhile, the drug companies continued to lose millions in business.

Despite the GAO's assertion the FDA wrongly used its AERs to launch an attack against ephedra, the general public still feared the herb ephedra due to mass media reports of its lethality. This fear of ephedra was used to mount yet another false attack against it in 2003.

Upon the death of Orioles Pitcher Steve Bechler, media quickly pointed to ephedra as the culprit. CBS News ran a story entitled *Ephedra Tied to Pitcher's Death* and reported the oft-repeated statement that it causes deaths, heart attacks and strokes. One critical point falsifies this statement. The ephedrine from ephedra had not yet been absorbed into Steve Bechler's body. According to Forensic pathologist Dr. Michael Baden, Former New York City chief medical examiner, in a letter to the Subcommittee on Oversight and Investigations Hearings on Issues Relating to Ephedra-Containing Dietary Supplements, July 23, 2003:

> "At the time Mr. Bechler collapsed from heat stroke, much of the ephedrine he had swallowed was still in his stomach and had not yet entered his blood stream. [The unabsorbed ephedrine] could not have caused or contributed to Mr. Bechler's death."[171]

Many professionals are quick to state that the ephedra elicited the heat stroke. A few key points falsify this statement as well. Bechler was using a supplement that contained a myriad of components, not just ephedra. How can you attribute negative side effects to just one herb when there were many consumed? Such an assumption could be made if previous clinical

---

[171] Fillon, Mike. *Ephedra Fact and Fiction.* Woodland Publishing. 2003. ISBN 1-58054-370-7.

trials pinpointed ephedra as the culprit in eliciting heat stroke. Yet, combining all the studies done on ephedra to date, not a single one has shown that heat stroke is a possible negative outcome associated with its use... not one!

In light of the controversy about the supposed link of ephedra to the tragic death of Steve Bechler, The Center for Exercise, Nutrition and Preventative Health Research (CENPHR) at Baylor University has provided insight as to the real causes of the heat stroke. According to their report, Mr. Bechler had a history of heat illness, hypertension and liver problems going all the way back to high school, had not eaten solid food for a day or two, was not acclimatized to training in the Florida heat, was wearing two to three layers of clothing during his workout, was already overweight, and was allowed by the Orioles personal trainer and medical doctor to exercise until he collapsed with a core temperature of 106° F.[172] Not wanting to take blame, it would appear as though the Orioles found ephedra to be their scapegoat.

Few Americans recognized the lazy reporting. Instead, they adhered to the media's often published doctrine that "Ephedra is good for nothing but killing you." Having the public on their side due to the Steve Bechler story, the FDA continued its campaign against ephedra utilizing the "RAND Report" to put on the final smack down.

Some background on the RAND Report: The National Institutes of Health commissioned the Rand Corporation to analyze public health issues surrounding the use of ephedra-containing products. This report was a meta-analysis of pub-

---

[172] Kreider, Richard. "The Alleged Role of Ephedra in the Death of a Professional Baseball Player." The Center for Exercise, Nutrition and Preventative Health Research (CENPHR) at Baylor University. February 21, 2003.

lished reports, journal articles, conference presentations and various sources of unpublished studies surrounding the use of ephedra and its effects. A meta-analysis is a quantitative approach to systematically combining the results of all previous research in order to arrive at a conclusion about a body of research.

The interpretations of the RAND Report by HHS and the FDA relative to the RAND report itself have glaring differences. In fact, well documented by Mike Fillon in his book, *Ephedra – Fact and Fiction*, it would appear that HHS and the FDA distorted the facts in their favor to eliminate their competitor from the market. Evidence of this can be seen by comparing the conclusion met by HHS and the FDA to the facts represented in the RAND Report. When compared, they are almost the antithesis of each other.

To clearly document the differences, we will quote the FDA's interpretation and the actual results published by RAND Corporation.

HHS and FDA: "...The study found limited evidence of an effect of ephedra on short-term weight loss, and minimal evidence of an effect on performance enhancement in certain physical activities."

RAND Report: "We combined the results of all studies in that group, using a statistical technique called meta-analysis, and calculated the average total weight lost as well as the average lost per month. Over the short term (four to six months), ephedrine, ephedrine plus caffeine, and supplements containing ephedra or ephedra plus caffeine promoted modest increases in weight loss, about two pounds per month more than the weight loss of persons taking the placebo. Products containing caffeine seemed to promote slightly more weight loss than those containing only ephedrine."

Hence, looking at numerous studies (via a meta-analysis), Rand Corporation found evidence that using ephedra elicited a loss in body fat of 2 pounds or more (depending on whether or not ephedra was used with caffeine) per month. Yet, according to the FDA, this is "limited evidence"? To the contrary, this is highly significant in that the average person could lose 12 pounds or more of fat over a period of 6 months. This is far better than any FDA approved fat loss drug such as Wellbutrin (Bupropion) or Meridia (sibutramine), where pharmaceutically funded trials showed a 5% loss in weight (not fat) at best. This creates a puzzle. How is it that 12 pounds of fat loss is not significant, yet a 5% loss in total weight, signifying an unhealthy loss in muscle, calls for FDA approval? The answer is simple: it doesn't.

Continuing, in the RAND Report, researchers of the Rand Corporation stated that "No studies have assessed the long-term effects of ephedra-containing dietary supplements or ephedrine on weight loss; the longest duration of treatment in a published study was six months." This is not true. As reported to the FDA by both Craig A. Molgaard, PhD, MPH, and the Proceedings of the 2002 International Congress on Obesity, a controlled clinical trial by Filozof et. al. entitled *The Effect of Ephedrine Plus Caffeine After a 4-week Portion Controlled Diet,* showed mean weight and waist-loss in the ephedrine/caffeine group that was significantly higher compared to the placebo group for up to one year of treatment."

The HHS and FDA further concluded that there was minimal evidence of an effect on performance enhancement in certain physical activities. This implies that the evidence was found which showed ephedra to have no effect on athletic performance. This is untrue. Simply, the only thing the RAND Report did state with respect to performance enhancement was the following:

Shane Ellison M.Sc.

"We found no studies that assessed the effects of ephedra-containing dietary supplements on athletic performance."

Hence, they could not find any studies that researched the
effect of ephedra on athletic performance. Further, they could
not find any evidence to show that ephedra use among athletes
was dangerous. This is strikingly different than concluding
that there was minimal evidence of an effect on performance
enhancement.

Continuing with half-truths, the FDA reported that the
RAND report found dangers associated with the use of ephedra.

HHS and FDA: "Ephedra is associated with higher risks
of mild to moderate side effects such as heart palpitations, psychiatric and upper gastrointestinal effects, and
symptoms of autonomic hyperactivity such as tremor and
insomnia, especially when it is taken with other stimulants."

Rand Corporation: "First, we reviewed the clinical trials
included in our analyses of weight loss and athletic performance, most of which reported adverse events for both
treatment and placebo groups. The trials contained no
reports of very serious adverse events (such as death and
cardiovascular events). This is not surprising, considering
that the occurrence of such events is likely to be quite rare
(less than one in a thousand users) and the clinical trials
included only a few thousand people."

The risk that the FDA was speaking of was about 0.1%. In
other words, of 1000 people who ingest ephedra or ephedrine,
1 might have an adverse effect. You are more likely to die from
a bee sting. West Virginia University estimates that 2 in 1000
people who get stung by bees die, making bee stings twice as

dangerous as ephedra (90-100 people dying every year). Even if you were to search high and low for an FDA drug that had such a positive safety profile as ephedra, you would not find it!

> HHS and FDA: "The study reviewed over 16,000 adverse events reported after ephedra use and found about 20 "sentinel events" including heart attack, stroke, and death that occurred in the absence of other contributing factors."

> RAND Corporation: "The majority of the adverse-event reports lacked sufficient information to demonstrate a connection between the event and use of ephedra or ephedrine. Nevertheless, we did identify a number of reports of sentinel and possible sentinel events, including death, stroke, myocardial infarction (heart attack), ventricular tachycardia/fibrillation, cardiac arrest, pulmonary arrest, transient ischemic attack, brain hemorrhage, seizure, psychiatric symptoms, and gastrointestinal symptoms."

According to this, the RAND Corporation scientists were unable to find any causal connection between consumption of ephedrine alkaloids and the adverse events reported by the FDA. The word sentinel, used by the RAND Corporation, HHS and FDA to describe some of the reported adverse events means that these events may indicate a safety hazard but do not prove that ephedra or ephedrine caused the adverse event.[173]

Still though, assuming that these events were caused by ephedra, it is hardly a cause for panic. As reported by USA Today, in 1999, the US government's Drug Abuse Warning Network counted 427 deaths from acetaminophen and 104

---

[173] Fillon, Mike. *Ephedra Fact and Fiction.* Woodland Publishing 2003. ISBN # 1-58054-370-7.

Shane Ellison M.Sc.

involving aspirin.[174] Perhaps the FDA should turn their attention to these over-the-counter painkillers that they have approved for use by children and adults alike. Moreover, perhaps professional football and baseball teams might want to ban the use of these frequently used substances, considering their ban of ephedra.

In summary to the RAND Report, despite the evidence showing ephedra and ephedrine to be safe, the analysis performed by RAND was an incomplete analysis of ephedra. With these flaws, one cannot technically use the report to make any kind of permanent decision regarding ephedra itself, we can only make inferences.

In their analysis, the RAND CORPORATION excluded valuable studies. Specifically, among the clinical trials where ephedra or ephedrine was used for weight loss, the investigators excluded over half (26 of 46) of the trials that have been performed. Most importantly, the Rand Corporation, being commissioned to analyze the natural plant ephedra, did not differentiate between ephedra and the pharmaceutical drug ephedrine. Among 20 trials used, only 5 involved the herbal ephedra-containing products.[175] Using two different compounds to make a conclusion on one is scientifically impossible. Either the FDA did not read the RAND Report in its entirely or they misunderstand scientific methodology, thereby not recognizing these flaws.

---

[174] Sullum, Jacob. "Ephedra no cause for panic." *USA Today*. McLean, VA. July 1, 2002. Page A11.

[175] Proposed Rule on Dietary Supplements Containing Ephedrine Alkaloids. FDA Docket No. 95N-0304.
Craig A. Molgaard, PhD, MPH, Professor and Acting Chair, Associate Dean for Research, Department of Preventive Medicine and Public Health, University of Kansas School of Medicine-Wichita, Comment to the FDA regarding Docket: 95N-0304-Dietary Supplements Containing Ephedrine Alkaloids.

Using the unfortunate death of Orioles Pitcher Steve Bechler as a catalyst and soliciting the help of the HHS to falsely interpret the RAND Report, the FDA won its battle against ephedra. On April 12, 2004, the sale of ephedra for use by Americans was prohibited. This ban was purported to be due to "unreasonable risk of illness or injury" when using ephedra.

An open letter to the Food and Drug Administration Commissioner Mark McClellan, M.D., Ph.D.

Dear Dr. McClellan,

As commissioner of the FDA you recently banned the natural plant ephedra for human consumption. Using the Dietary Supplement Health and Education Act (DSHEA) of 1994, you have successfully leveraged your power to convince Americans that this dietary supplement presents a significant or unreasonable risk of illness or injury when used properly. Amazingly, you did this by paying the RAND Corporation to publish a study showing the immediate danger of ephedra. Never mind that the report would have failed a freshman level science course for its blatant lack of scientific method such as excluding over half of the known trials in their analysis and not differentiating between the plant ephedra and the synthetic drug ephedrine. Still though, using the report, you did a great job of convincing medical doctors that this natural herb, which has been used successfully for over 5000 years in Asian medicine, is good for nothing but killing people.

You have not only perverted the truth, but also made a historic, hypocritical attack on dietary supplements, which have killed fewer people than bee stings. Sadly, we cannot say the same for your "FDA Approved" drugs, which, ac-

---

cording to the *Journal of the American Medical Association* kill approximately 300 people per day![176]

Your hypocrisy is derived from the fact that Americans can still obtain an "APPROVED," yet inferior form of ephedra from their doctor, which is a man-made version known as ephedrine HCl. Moreover, they can also obtain it for their children via over-the-counter cough syrup, which contains another inferior form known as pseudoephedrine! Lacking the entire spectrum of ingredients found in their natural form and being absorbed at a much faster and harmful rate than their natural counterpart, your approved drugs are proven to be more dangerous than ephedra. Yet you have approved them for use by children!

This is ridiculous to argue about safety and efficacy. This is not about safety and efficacy, it's about money! After all, According to *USA Today*, over half of the experts you hire have direct financial relationships with the pharmaceutical companies who are losing BILLIONS of dollars from the sales of ephedra knock-offs. Oh, I stand corrected, who WERE losing billions of dollars.

You even went as far as RAIDING numerous ephedra suppliers and stealing thousands of dollars worth of products from their shelves! You defended this unconstitutional act by stating:

"Consumers must have accurate and truthful health information so they can make informed choices, and the FDA will continue its aggressive enforcement efforts against companies that make misleading claims about their products."

[176] Lucian Leape. "Error in medicine." *Journal of the American Medical Association*, 1994, 272:23, p 1851. Also: Leape LL. Institute of Medicine medical error figures are not exaggerated. *Journal of the American Medical Association*. 2000 Jul 5;284(1):95-7.

Are you serious? Your cohorts in the pharmaceutical industry have been making "misleading claims" in their drug marketing ads since 1997 and you have not done a SINGLE thing to stop them! In fact, they spend 2-3 billion dollars annually to not just spread lies, but DAMN lies about their man made drugs. Your only action has been a simple letter recommending that they change their ads. You never once stole their products. And you never once filed charges for their blatant disregard for the Food, Drug, and Cosmetic Act (FFDCA) Act, which clearly states that drug ads cannot be false and misleading.

Your hypocrisy is never ending. The FDA as an organization is filled with deliberate, objectively demonstrable lies and highly misleading half-truths. Worse, the FDA has completely avoided whole truths with regards to ephedra. Considering that your FDA approved drugs kill about 100,000 Americans per year, I vote not to ban ephedra but rather ban the FDA. Perhaps this will become a reality as more people awaken to your hypocrisy and the corruption of the FDA.

Shane Ellison, M.Sc.
www.healthmyths.net
healthmyths@safe-mail.net

The bottom line is that Americans have been fraudulently convinced that ephedra is dangerous. The strongest support for this assertion comes from conclusions met by accredited scientists who have relentlessly studied the effects of ephedra, not ephedrine, and its safety via scientifically sound, controlled clinical trials. These studies have not only looked at the safety of ephedra but also whether or not the herb induces heart attack, stroke, and seizures. To ensure that there are no misinterpretations, the conclusions met by scientists are often quoted below in their entirety.

Craig A. Molgaard, PhD, MPH, of the Department of Preventive Medicine and Public Health at University of Kansas School of Medicine-Wichita submitted Comment to the FDA regarding the ephedra ban. With an extensive background in epidemiology, he concluded that:

> "Despite the extensive use of ephedra alkaloids in the United States, with hundreds of millions of caplets sold annually, we note no controlled epidemiologic studies that support an association between ingestion of ephedra alkaloids, whether ingested alone or with caffeine, and stroke, seizure, or myocardial infarction. We know of no evidence, with hundreds of millions of caplets sold annually, of increases in the rates of those diseases in the U.S. population. In fact, those rates are either stable or declining."

> "The controlled clinical trials with ephedrine involve hundreds of subjects. Yet, none of the studies has reported significant adverse events. More importantly, none of the studies has included a single subject who experienced stroke, seizure, or myocardial infarction while consuming ephedra alkaloids, despite treatments for as long as twelve months. Clinical trials such as those of Boozer (2001 and 2002) and Astrup (1986, 1990, 1991, 1992, 1995) are scientifically sound."[177]

Specific to the issue of whether or not ephedra causes stroke, Yale Researchers posted their assertive findings in the peer-reviewed journal *Neurology*:

---

[177] Craig A. Molgaard, PhD, MPH, Professor and Acting Chair Associate Dean for Research, Department of Preventive Medicine and Public Health, University of Kansas School of Medicine-Wichita. Comment to the FDA regarding Docket: 95N-0304-*Dietary Supplements Containing Ephedrine Alkaloids*. 02-28-2003.

"Ephedra is not associated with increased risk for hemorrhagic stroke, except possibly at higher doses."[178]

Almost as if reprimanding the FDA, Attorneys-at-Law Jonathan W. Emord, Claudia A. Lewis-Eng, and Kathryn E. Balmford for Emord and Associates, P.C. state:

"The Joint Commenters have shown that the Proposed Rule [regarding the ban of ephedra] lacks a scientific foundation in empirically valid data. They have shown that the agency has not met its burden of proof under 21 U.S.C. § 343(f) (the adulteration standard for dietary supplements) to justify removing ephedrine alkaloid-containing dietary supplements from the market or to justify the Proposed Rule. The Joint Commenters have shown that the Proposed Rule is arbitrary and capricious, contrary to law, and violates the First Amendment, and the Joint Commenters have offered FDA a scientifically valid alternative in the form of a 25 mg/serving; 90 mg/day ephedrine alkaloid limit and a reasonable disclaimer substantially indistinguishable from the one now used on ephedrine and pseudoephedrine-containing over-the-counter drugs. To ensure compliance with all applicable law and to protect the public health, the Joint Commenters urge FDA to adopt the alternative to its Proposed Rule that they recommend herein."[179]

USA Today made their voice heard as well. Understanding that the FDA's Adverse Event Reports failed to associate the use of ephedra with negative outcomes, Reporter Jacob

---

[178] Yale University. *Neurology* 2003. 60:132-135.

[179] Jonathan W. Emord, Claudia A. Lewis-Eng, Kathryn E. Balmford for E M O R D & A S S O C I A T E S, P.C., ATTORNEYS-AT –LAW, CONSTITUTIONAL AND ADMINISTRATIVE LAW, to FDA Docket No. 95N-0304.

Sullum is quick to clarify this deceitful use of statistics to the public by making it known that:

> "The professional alarmists at *Public Citizen* count well over 100 deaths reported to the FDA (among) people using ephedra-containing products since 1993. It's worth noting that a 2000 *New England Journal of Medicine* study found that fewer than a third of the adverse events supposedly caused by ephedra were definitely or probably related to the use of the drug."[180]

Among one of the largest studies ever performed on the use of ephedra was a collaborative effort by the New York Obesity Research Center, St. Luke's-Roosevelt Hospital and Columbia University; Beth Israel-Deaconess Medical Center, Harvard Medical School; CIGNA health care; and Vanderbilt University Medical Center. These researchers investigated the effects of ingesting 90 mg of ephedra with 192 mg of caffeine daily for a duration of six months. Shockingly, these researchers, among the most respected in the world, found that this herbal supplement reduced body weight by up to 11 pounds and body fat while at the same time decreasing LDL-cholesterol levels and increasing HDL-cholesterol levels significantly. With respect to negative side effects it was noted that, "There were no significant adverse effects resulting from treatment with herbal ephedra/caffeine in the present study."[181] This is in huge contrast to what the FDA has reported.

Recognizing that this went against the adverse event reports collected and reported by the FDA, researchers C.N. Boozer and colleagues asked, "How can the absence of treatment-related adverse events in this and two previous clinical trials of ephedra combinations (334 subjects total) be recon-

---

[180] Jacob Sullum. *USA Today*. McLean, Va.: July 1, 2002. Page A11.
[181] Boozer, C.N. et al. *International Journal of Obesity*. 2002. 26. 593-604.

ciled with the adverse event reports collected by the FDA for users of these products?" The explanations proposed included coincidence, pre-existing conditions, non-recommended usage, and individual sensitivity. In other words, those who were already sick and destined to have a negative health affect consumed ephedra and blamed the eventual worsening health on ephedra. Or, irresponsible people used exorbitant dosages; similarly, an alcoholic dies from over consumption of alcohol. These variables can never be controlled and as such do not constitute the prohibition of a natural medicine with such health benefits.

Scientists from across the ocean have reached similar conclusions. Soren Toubro and colleagues from the Research Department of Human Nutrition in Denmark studied the effects of using 60 mg of ephedra and 200 mg of caffeine daily for six months. Their conclusion, like all other controlled clinical trials, is in sharp contrast to those met by the FDA. "We conclude that the ephedrine/caffeine combination is safe and effective in long-term treatment in improving and maintaining weight loss. The side effects are minor and transient and no clinically relevant withdrawal symptoms have been observed."[182]

If ephedra were dangerous, it would be safe to assume that its so-called devastating effects would be seen in children. Still though, research looking at the effects of ephedra and caffeine use among adolescents has proven that ephedra is safe for kids. As published in the *International Journal of Obesity*, we find that children who used as little as 30 mg of ephedra and 300 mg of caffeine were able to lose an average of 17 pounds of fat while those obese children not consuming the herbal preparation lost a mere 1 pound! With respect to negative side effects, it was reported by the scientists that the total number of side

---

[182] Toubro, S. et al. *International Journal of Obesity Related Metabolic Disorders*. 1993 Dec; 17 Suppl 3:s73-7; discussion s82.

effects among those taking the herbal preparation and those not taking it were not different. They also noted that the small number of side effects reported subsided after consistent use of the herbal preparation.[183]

Childhood obesity is rampant in the US, mainly due to excessive use of sugar. Carol Torgan, PhD, writing for the National Institutes of Health, has stated that childhood obesity has doubled over the last two to three decades, causing 1 in 5 children to be overweight! It would seem that these findings would present an exciting avenue by which doctors could essentially cure this epidemic while at the same time, wipe out the afflictions associated with being obese, such as diabetes.

More than protecting our right to ephedra, this chapter elucidates the importance of protecting our rights to natural medicine as a means of procuring our health. Letting the FDA ban ephedra has opened the door for future attack on safe and effective natural medicines that serve as competitors to pharmaceutical drugs. Next on the hit list are such herbs as Kava Kava, Glucosamine Sulfate, Yohimbe, St. John's Wort, Gingko Biloba and Citrus Aurantium just to name a few.

Shortly after the banning of ephedra, Consumer Reports was commissioned to run a story entitled, *Dangerous supplements: Still at large.* Once again, lazy reporting and anecdotal reports of major health problems attributed to the use various herbs dominated science and logic. A few more stories with fearful titles and Americans will be begging the FDA to ban safe and effective herbs, thereby reducing their chances of obtaining health to an even smaller proportion.

With the success of the ephedra ban, the FDA knows they can successfully scare the American population into thinking a

---

[183] Molnar D. et al. *International Journal of Obesity.* 2000. 24, 1573-1578.

given natural medicine is dangerous and thereby gain support for the banning of it when it poses competition to the pharmaceutical industry. This guarantees that America remains one Nation, under Drugs, indivisible, with perceived liberty and sickness for all. To remedy this, health consumers must become self-educated on the proper use of natural medicine and begin to inform others of its benefits, including congressmen.

Myth #10 – Dieting is the Cure for Obesity

Fact – Those who adhere to the outdated model of treating obesity by dieting will have continued fat gain followed by worsening health in their later years.

Globally, obesity has reached epidemic proportions. More than 1 billion adults are overweight. At least 300 million of them are clinically obese. Obesity is a major contributor to the global burden of chronic disease and disability, often leading to Type-II diabetes, cardiovascular disease, hypertension and stroke, as well as certain forms of cancer.

Fat loss is the single most important step toward obtaining health and longevity. Therefore, the cause and cure of obesity, typically defined as having a Body Mass Index (BMI) of over 25, demands attention. If a weight issue is not addressed, all other preventative health measures are null and void, period.

Recognizing the importance of being thin and fit, millions of Americans are on the latest and greatest fad diet. Whether it is their physician or personal trainer, Americans are barraged with the oft-repeated statement "go on a diet." This is all for naught, as Americans are consistently among the fattest people in the world.

The obesity problem in America has surged to epidemic proportions. According to the National Institutes of Health, two-thirds of US adults are overweight. Moreover, approximately 800 Americans will die from obesity today.

Rather than recognize that perhaps dieting and exercise is not the answer, obese people are often mislabeled as being lazy, or worse, referred to as "pigs." This is simply untrue; their only crime would be failing to search for the true cause of obesity and incorporating what they learned into their exercise and eating plan. While obscured, it is not totally hidden.

Pushing aside the outdated model of eating less and exercising more, millions of obese individuals have medical research to turn to that unravels the obesity mystery. Once unraveled, it is discovered that both adults and children alike, even in the rare instance that it may be due to genetics, can in fact, overcome obesity. Before disclosing the often-missed principles of fat loss, it is important to learn the cause of obesity. By analyzing the cause, the cure and the shortcomings of dieting become evident.

Sifting through decades of scientific research on obesity, it is learned that fat loss has little to do with dieting, and in many cases, exercising, too. But you don't have to be a rocket scientist to recognize this. We have all met or know of someone who eats whatever they want on a daily basis, yet fails to gain fat. Conversely, we also know someone who eats sensibly, but seems to gain more weight every year, eventually becoming overtly obese.

In many cases, obesity is the result of an inactive sympathetic nervous system.[184] Stick with this definition, while it sounds a bit complex, its meaning will be simplified. This

---

[184] Bray, GA. "Obesity, a disorder of nutrient partitioning: the MONA LISA hypothesis." *Journal of Nutrition.* 1991 Aug; 121(8):1146-62.

cause of obesity has become so apparent that scientists from Harvard, Columbia, New York Obesity Research Center, and the Research Dept. of Human Nutrition in Copenhagen, Denmark have coined the phrase MONA LISA to describe it.[185] MONA LISA stands for Most Obesities kNown are Low In Sympathetic Activity. In simpler terms, MONA LISA means that obese people have lost their natural ability to burn fat due to lack of activity of the sympathetic nervous system. This may be due to genetics, high sugar intake, aging, a sedentary lifestyle, or a combination of factors.

The sympathetic nervous system controls a wide range of biological functions required to keep us alive. With respect to obesity, it utilizes chemicals known as adrenaline and nor-adrenaline released from the adrenal glands to activate the fat burning mechanism known as "adaptive thermogenesis," or thermogenesis for short.

Thermogenesis has been considered your God-given right to be thin.[186] It is the process by which excess calories consumed are converted to heat rather than stored as fat. Thermogenesis occurs in Brown Adipose Tissue (BAT) when the sympathetic nervous system (with adrenaline and noradrenaline) ignites BAT via β-receptors. This ability of BAT is obviously unique. In most cells, mitochondria (considered the powerhouse of the cell) use the energy they liberate to make the energy-producing molecule ATP (adenosine triphosphate) that is converted to "work." ATP is the fuel that drives chemical reactions in living organisms and allows you to have the energy to run on a treadmill. In BAT however, the protein UCP-1 (uncoupling protein 1) interferes with this process, forcing the cells of BAT to release the energy as heat instead of ATP. This is why fat can

---

[185] Boozer, CN. Et al. *International Journal of Obesity.* 2002. 26. 593-604.

[186] Mowrey, Daniel. *Fat Management – The Thermogenic Factor.* ISBN 0-93626-107-2.

be burned while sitting at the dinner table instead of running on the treadmill. Heat production does not require work, but ATP production does. The phenomenon of releasing energy as heat instead of work has been termed mitochondrial proton "leak," and is solely dependent on UCP-1.

In addition to igniting thermogenesis in BAT, the sympathetic nervous system also ignites lipolysis in white adipose tissue, typically found in the abdominal and hip region. Lipolysis mobilizes fat (triglycerides) into the bloodstream for utilization as fuel.

In agreement with the MONA LISA hypothesis, it has been found that heat production is greater among lean individuals, whereas the obese have very little heat production after a meal.[187] This explains in part why some people can eat whatever they want and never gain fat while others seem to gain fat simply by looking at food.

In summarizing this process, just as diabetics do not release insulin, the obese do not release enough ADRENALINE or NORADRENALINE to activate thermogenesis among BAT. BAT protects against diet-induced obesity by burning excess calories consumed via thermogenesis.[188] As a result, instead of burning fat, they store it and their body uses carbohydrates and amino acids as fuel. Over time, they will continue to gain more fat, regardless of diet and exercise.

Needless to say, activating thermogenesis among the obese is the Holy Grail for burning fat. Through the complicated

[187] Thorne, A. et al. "Meal-induced thermogenesis in obese patients before and after weight reduction." *Clinical Physiology.* 1989 Oct;9(5):481-98.

[188] Hamman, A. et al. "Decreased brown fat markedly enhances susceptibility to diet induced obesity, diabetes, and hyperlipidemia." *Endocrinology.* 1996 Jan;137(1):21-9

"thermogenic cascade," the sum result of activating thermogenesis is increased fat loss. If a person wants to lose fat and remain healthy, they must understand the activation of thermogenesis.

Utilizing exercise to activate thermogenesis is difficult. Specifically, an individual would have to work out for 1.5 to 4 hours in order to turn on the natural fat furnace through exercise![189] This is why endurance athletes do not have a problem with obesity and why lifting weights and fad diets rarely have an effect on fat loss.

Limiting caloric intake by dieting wreaks havoc on thermogenesis. To clarify this we can look to prescription drugs and yo-yo dieting. Most prescription drugs for fat loss work to decrease appetite. A drug that weakens the appetite or curbs it not only weakens the immune system, but also will cause any weight that was lost to come back once the user quits the drug.

This is not inexplicable. Thermogenesis is activated by food intake. This is termed Diet-Induced Thermogenesis (DIT). Therefore, when a person decreases food intake, thermogenesis is "down regulated" to accommodate for the lack of caloric intake. Once the person begins to eat normal again, they will be feeding a body that lacks normal thermogenesis. As a result, the excess calories consumed cannot be turned into heat and are instead stored as fat.

This same principle applies to dieting as well, which is why it rarely or temporarily works. Everybody has noticed this phenomenon, as can be seen by the coined term "yo-yo" dieting.

---

[189] Rhoades and Pflanzer. *Human Physiology.* Third Edition. ISBN# 0-03-005159-2.

Recognizing the inadequacies of exercise, prescription drugs and limiting caloric intake by dieting to curb the obesity epidemic, our own attitudes and ways of thinking must change. In doing so, we must adhere to what science has shown with relation to MONA LISA, thermogenesis and obesity.

To do this we can live by 5 principles that activate thermogenesis. This is not about fad diets, magic pills or fantasy claims to transform the way you look overnight. These principles are based on accurate, scientific information that can help both adults and children who suffer from MONA LISA effectively change the way their body responds to food. These principles are not one-time principles but rather a lifetime change. Considering the ease at which these principles can be applied and their efficacy for shedding the fat, they could rightly be called the "Lazy Man's Guide to Fat Loss."

Principle 1 – Eat 4-6 Meals Per Day

Rather than reduce caloric intake, one should feed their body 4-6 healthy meals per day. To keep it simple, healthy means consuming proteins, low glycemic index carbohydrates, and essential fatty acids, while eliminating sweets and juice. This guarantees that you do not lower your body's thermogenic capabilities while at the same time ensuring that thermogenesis stays active all day long, as juice and sweets block thermogenesis.

To simplify even further, it could be noted that by drinking water with meals instead of soda or juice, while eliminating anything "sweet," a person would gain significant benefits as seen by continued fat loss, especially children.

There is no single eating plan that is right for everyone. Every individual has a unique metabolism. To learn about your options, a few authors come to mind. Most notably, they are Barry Sears, Dr. Joseph Mercola and Jay Robb. Reading books by these authors will educate you on basic food science and give you a wide range of options to choose from with respect to eating plans. Ultimately, this will allow you to personalize your meal planning and find an eating plan that's right for you. First, keep it simple my eliminating soda, juice, and sweets from your meals. This simple approach will make a big difference.

Principle 2 – Use a Thermogenic Aid

The term Thermogenic Aid has become synonymous with fat burning. As a result, any products with this word on the label seem to sell themselves. Unfortunately, very few fulfill the promise.

A true Thermogenic ignites thermogenesis and can have lasting effects without having to depend on them for life. While exciting, true thermogens are far and few between, especially in light of the ephedra ban. It's important to note, a Thermogenic Aid is not for everyone and should only be used when all other routes of fat loss have been exhausted.

Decades ago, it was found that one could activate thermogenesis and thereby stimulate brown fat activity through the consumption of certain substances in the diet. The most effective of these substances was ephedra. As research advanced, utilizing a blend of ephedra and caffeine or ephedra, caffeine, and aspirin enhanced the effectiveness and safety of ephedra.

The EC or ECA stacks are considered "sympathomimetics" because they mimic adrenaline and noradrenaline by activating β-receptors of the adrenergic system. This activation sparks the thermogenic cascade as well as inhibits the body's ability to shut it down. Additionally, the stack decreases the minor negative side effects of a thermogenic agent, such as jitters and short half-life. These stacks have been proven time and again to be safe and effective at curing obesity. Controlled studies substantiate this, as can be seen in the aforementioned material discussing ephedra safety.

Because ephedra carries so much political heat and controversy, supplement makers were quick to discover and produce alternatives to the EC and ECA stack. While difficult, it is not impossible to find a fat burning replacement to these stacks. Success was dependent on finding an herb that, like ephedra, targeted β-receptors of the adrenergic system. Remember, the sympathetic nervous system naturally activates these receptors using adrenaline and noradrenaline.

Relying on Chinese medicine once again, a safe and effective replacement to ephedra has commonly been Zhi Shi (*Citrus aurantium*). In 2002, Georgetown University Medical Center asserted that Zhi Shi might be the best thermogenic substitute to ephedra.[190]

According to researchers at McGill University, Zhi Shi contains a molecular cousin to ephedrine known as phenylephrine as well as N-methyl-tyramine, hordenine, octaopamine, and tyramine. Because they activate the adrenergic system (which is responsible for activating thermogenesis) these compounds are known as adrenergic amines.[191]

The most notable adrenergic amine is phenylephrine. Not as strong as ephedrine, it must be used under two conditions to be effective. First, researchers have found that its quantity of phenylephrine must be boosted to equal 30% rather than 2%. Anything less than 30% is typically ineffective at burning

---

[190] Preuss, H.G. et al. "Citrus aurantium as a thermogenic, weight reduction replacement for ephedra: an overview." *Journal of Medicine.* 2002;33(1-4):247-64.

[191] Fontana, E. et al. "Effects of octaopamine on lipolysis, glucose transport and amine oxidation in mammalian fat cells." *Comparative Biochemistry and Physiology C-Pharmacology, Toxicology and Endocrinology.* 2000 Jan;125(1):33-44.

fat. Secondly, similar to ephedra, phenylephrine from Zhi Shi must be mixed with a conglomeration of supporting herbs. Such herbs may include but are not limited to green tea catechins, ginger, aspirin, cayenne, synthetic caffeine, guarana, and Yohimbe extracts. If the herbs are chosen properly and used in the proper amount and ratio relative to other herbs, the thermogenic product will inhibit the body's ability to shut down thermogenesis prematurely.

Without meeting these two criteria, Zhi Shi, even a 30% extract, will not afford the user any fat loss. Therefore, while Zhi Shi is becoming well known, few companies will harness its true fat burning abilities, as they will typically use standard Zhi Shi rather than an extract. Naturally, Zhi Shi only contains 2-3% phenylephrine. This is hardly enough to have an effect on fat loss.

Currently, a supplement known as Ephedra Free ThermoFX is among the most potent natural supplements available. Real life applications have shown unprecedented success in helping those who suffer from MONA LISA shed fat. It can be found at www.health-fx.net.

Principle 3 – Just say No to Sugar and Artificial Flavors

Boldly put, sugar (sucrose and concentrated fructose) is the number one contributing factor to poor health and premature aging. Whiter than cocaine and deadlier than any illicit drug, sugar could rightfully be considered the silent killer sitting in your kitchen. That sugar is dangerous remains below the radar of health professionals and as such remains the biggest health secret of all time.

In addition to making you look 10 years older, sugar consumption leads to diabetes, depression, osteoporosis, cancer[192] (increases your risk of suffering from lung cancer by 28%) and heart disease. Adding to the list, the World Health Organization (WHO) officially announced that sugar also contributes to obesity.

That sugar greatly increases obesity will rarely be publicized. Furious over the claim made by the WHO, the sugar industry threatened to "challenge" the $460 million funding given to the WHO by the United States for making this "dubious" claim.

Don't let the lack of media behind sugars ill effects deter you from understanding the implications of its use. Sugar is so detrimental to fat loss that healthy eating and exercise rarely has any effect on obesity among those who consume sugar through soda, diet soda, candy, chocolate, cereal, health food bars, sugar fortified protein shakes and ice cream.

Let's look at the truth behind sugar. When sugar, or to be specific, sucrose, is consumed, it elicits a corresponding overproduction and release of the hormone insulin. The pancreas secretes insulin. Typically, insulin is secreted in relatively small amounts when proteins, carbohydrates and fats are consumed. Insulin's main job is to sweep the previously mentioned nutrients into the cell for energy and ultimately, growth. To this end, insulin binds to a receptor on the surface of cells. This allows the entry of glucose, fatty acids and amino acids into cells such as muscle and fat cells. Once inside, these nutrients are converted to glycogen, triglycerides and proteins, respectively. In addition to these actions, insulin is also a potent stimulator of growth factors, including insulin-growth factor 1 (IGF-1).

---

[192] Registro Nacional De Cancer, Montevideo, Uraguay. Dietary sugar and lung cancer: a case control study in Uraguay. *Nutr Cancer.* 1998:31(2):132-7.

Insulin also inhibits catabolic processes such as the breakdown of glycogen and fat, and decreases the production of glucose from lactate and amino acids (gluconeogenesis). From the actions of insulin, we can see that it serves several very important, life-sustaining roles as an anabolic hormone due to its ability to stimulate growth.

Noticeably, insulin is not all bad. Problems arise when insulin is released in abnormally high amounts in response to sugar. We will call this the "insulin spike." The insulin spike is the result of sugar's fast absorption into the blood stream relative to fructose and other food. Understanding the detrimental effects of the insulin spike on obesity will hopefully deter us from consuming sugar.

The insulin spike greatly inhibits our body's ability to burn excess calories by turning off thermogenesis. Simply put, the overflow of insulin causes our body to tell fat cells to store, store, store, while it tells your brain to eat, eat, eat. More accurately, the insulin spike from sugar inhibits hormone-sensitive lipase (HSL) while promoting the activity of lipoprotein lipase. By inhibiting HSL the body is no longer able to release triglycerides (fat) into the bloodstream to be used for fuel consumption, thereby resulting in the storage of fat.[193] When HSL is activated from the spike in insulin, triglycerides that have previously been released into the bloodstream are removed and deposited back into fat cells. The sum result is an increase in abdominal fat storage.

Children are not immune to this effect. *Lancet* reported that scientists have found that children who consume even a single soda per day are 60% more likely to become obese.[194]

---

[193] Roduit, Raphael. *A role for hormone-sensitive lipase in glucose-stimulated Insulin secretion: a study in hormone-sensitive lipase-deficient mice.*

[194] *The Lancet.* 2001;357:505-508.

In addition to storing fat, sugar users overeat. Those who consume sugar are often unable to know when they have eaten too much and unconsciously go on an eating binge. This is due to the insulin spike, which results in a subsequent drop. This drop will make us feel artificially hungry. To curb this sensation of hunger, the sugar user will typically reach for more sugar or other source of food to satisfy it. This inevitably leads to over feeding and fat gain.

Professor Terry Davidson and associate professor Susan Withers at Purdue University have discovered that artificial sweeteners, like sugar, disrupt satiety, the feeling of being full. Their results, published in *International Journal of Obesity* showed that "mouth feel" plays a crucial role in the body's ability to count calories and that when we consume artificial sweeteners, we disrupt the body's ability to count calories based on sweetness. Thus, artificial sweeteners cause us to overeat without conscious awareness.[195] In other words, you think you're not eating like a pig, but in reality you are.

Apparently, makers of health food bars and protein supplements have not been made aware of the ill effects of sugar. This can be seen by the fact that most every health food bar and protein supplement is loaded with sugar or artificial sweeteners. The belief that these bars and supplements are healthy for you is a perfect example of how marketing strategies can supersede medical science and common sense.

Instead of "low carb" we need low or no sugar. Recognizing this, a SafeTaste© Certification has been employed to act as a regulatory measure among health foods and supplements. Yielding the SafeTaste© Certification shows consumers that in fact the health food or supplement they are consuming

---

[195] Davidson, T.L. and Swithers, S.E. "A Pavlovian approach to the problem of obesity." *International Journal of Obesity Related Metabolic Disorders.* 2004 Jul;28(7):933-5.

contains no sugar (sucrose) or artificial flavors. Without this certification, be wary of consuming it, as they will elicit the negative responses mentioned here, regardless of what the label reads.

Learn more at www.safetastecertification.com.

Repeated use of sugar leads to multiple insulin spikes and over time, insulin receptors become desensitized. Inevitably, this leads to a disorder known as insulin resistance. As a result, glucose, and other nutrients, is not able to make its journey into the cells of the body where it can be used as fuel and remains in the bloodstream. Insulin resistance leads to obesity in the following ways:

- Less glucose is converted to energy causing it to be stored as fat.

- Since your body isn't converting food to energy properly, it demands more food. As a result, sugar cravings increase, as does excessive eating and binge eating.

- Lack of energy production leads to fatigue.

- As insulin resistance and weight gain continue to increase, your body further loses its ability to process foods correctly, causing even MORE weight gain.

Of paramount importance, medical doctors often mistake insulin resistance as diabetes. This err in diagnoses stems from the fact that both conditions cause excessive blood glucose levels when fasting. Commonly, this is perceived as lack of insulin, since insulin is responsible for clearing the bloodstream of glucose. In reality though, there is plenty of insulin. The problem lies in the fact that the body has simply become insensitive to it.

Rather than striving to reverse insulin resistance, this err in diagnoses leads to the use of insulin by patients. Hence, introducing more insulin to the already insulin resistant body compounds the problem. As a result, insulin resistance becomes amplified and cells are no longer able to take up vital nutrients. This triggers a massive loss in nutrients such as B vitamins, magnesium, zinc, essential amino acids, carbohydrates and proteins. Not able to make it into the cell due to insulin resistance, essential nutrients, as well as glucose, are simply excreted in the urine.

Essentially, insulin resistance shuts your body off from receiving life enhancing nutrients. Over time, the heart, kidneys, peripheral nerves and your eyes, just to name a few, begin to shut down.

In a few instances, insulin resistance does lead to diabetes. Because the pancreas cannot continually secrete insulin, it becomes exhausted and shuts down; this is termed type-2 diabetes. For health and longevity it is imperative that insulin resistance and diabetes are differentiated. This will allow for proper treatment rather than compounding the problem of insulin resistance.

Of further importance, both insulin resistance and diabetes greatly increase ones chances of suffering from a heart attack. Researchers claim that men with diabetes are two to four times more likely to experience a heart attack or stroke relative to a person without the disease and women two to six times more likely.[196] It would be safe to say that these same statistics apply to those with insulin resistance, as the culprit in the increased risk of heart disease is an elevated level of glucose in the bloodstream.

---

[196] *Annals of Internal Medicine.* April 20, 2004;140: 644-649.

The mechanism by which glucose causes heart disease demands your full attention. Not being able to gain entry into the cell, excess glucose remains in the blood stream and undergoes a chemical process known as oxidation. This process was discovered as far back as 1912 by the french chemist L. Maillard. This oxidation results in a glucose derivative referred to as advanced glycation end products or AGE-products. Like a knife carving clay, AGE-products scar arterial walls. The scarring results in plague buildup. The excessive plaque buildup will eventually clog the arteries, leading to heart attack or stroke.

To circumvent the negative results of insulin resistance and diabetes, glucose must be cleared from the bloodstream. Aside from quitting sugar, several nutrients must be consumed on a regular basis and in the proper dosage. To mention a few they are alpha-lipoic acid, acetyl-L-carnitine, whey protein isolate, green tea extract, steviosides (from stevia extract) and vanadyl sulfate.

In total, sugar is a deadly obesity trap. Internalize this. The negative effects of excess insulin released due to the consumption of sugar can occur temporarily, or worse, in the case of insulin resistance, permanently alter a person's metabolism in a negative manner. Over time, sugar consumption will undoubtedly cause you to become a slave to an out-of-control biochemical nightmare that never ends, all the while causing you to gain more fat, age prematurely (as seen through aged skin) and bring you closer to an early death.

Sugar is simply not designed for the human metabolism. Resultantly, very few substances wreak more havoc on our health than sugar, yet the average American consumes about 150 pounds of sugar annually.[197]

---

[197] Leighton, Steward. et al. *The New Sugar Busters! Cut Sugar to Trim Fat.* ISBN 0-345-46958-5.

Shane Ellison M.Sc.

This brings us to the inevitable topic of quitting sugar. Quitting sugar will be the least popular principle among sugar addicts. Not only does sugar taste good but it is also physically addicting. Without it, regular users are often irritable, hungry and lack focus. However, by slowing weaning one's self from sugar, ex-sugar addicts will be ecstatic to learn of their new-found reward of health and longevity. This will be manifested into endless energy, elevated mood and appetite control. In fact, it is not a stretch to say that over time, quitting sugar will make you look and feel 10 years younger. So, rather than focus on devising a complex diet and exercise plan, one should first plan on how to quit consuming sugar and artificial flavors. While implementing this plan, healthy eating and exercise can be added to your healthy living endeavors.

A sweet tip for quitting sugar is to use natural alternatives to sugar such as stevia extract. Stevia extract has been used for over 20 years in Japan and Brazil. Not only does stevia extract taste great but it also does not inhibit thermogenesis, lead to insulin resistance or diabetes. To add to the benefits of stevia extract, previous animal and human studies show that stevia extract lowers systolic and diastolic blood pressure, prevents as well as reverses insulin resistance, and works to clear glucose from the blood stream by up to 30%.[198] This is phenomenal to say the least.

In light of the discoveries made about stevia extract, the word sugar should be replaced with the word stevia in every

[198] Hsieh, M.H. et al. "Efficacy and tolerability of oral stevioside in patients with mild essential hypertension: A two-year, randomized, placebo-controlled study." *Clinical Therapy.* 2003 Nov;25(11):2797-808.
Lailerd, N. et al. "Effects of stevioside on glucose transport activity in insulin-sensitive and insulin –resistant rat skeletal muscle." *Metabolism.* 2004 Jan;53(1):101-7.
Gregerson, S. et al. "Antihyperglucemic effects of stevioside in type 2 diabetic subjects." *Metabolism.* 2004 Jan;53(1):73-6.

household. Stevia can be purchased at a local health food store and used to sweeten anything such as coffee, tea, or desserts.

Adding to sweet tips for dissolving the sugar habit we look to the use of L-tryptophan. Sugar cravings have been associated with low levels of serotonin, thereby causing irritability, hunger and lack of focus. As serotonin drops, we crave sugar. To deter this biochemical imbalance and avoid sugar cravings, we can supplement with the essential amino acid L-tryptophan (not 5-hydroxy-L-tryptophan). L-tryptophan is a chemical precursor to serotonin. When consumed, it raises serotonin levels in the brain. This will ensure that serotonin levels remain constant and therefore halt the uncontrollable urge to eat sugar.

Diet Coke is a Joke

Countless numbers of dieters consume Diet Coke thinking that it is inert to their diet efforts. After all, it's called Diet Coke, right? Wrong! Diet Coke, regardless of how many calories it has, wreaks havoc on your diet efforts and will ultimately cause you to gain weight.

When it comes to losing fat, it is more about how much sugar (or sugar substitute) you consume rather than calories or dietary fat intake. Hence, the goal is to consume as little sugar as possible (including fruits and their juices). Why? The sweet flavor elicits the release of insulin from the pancreas to enhance the uptake of sugar by the cells so that it doesn't linger in the bloodstream. Once insulin is released it inhibits your fat burning hormone called "hormone sensitive lipase" (HSL). This hormone is responsible for releasing fat into the bloodstream to be utilized as fuel. If inhibited, your body is unable to burn fat and will then begin utilizing amino acids (from muscle) and carbohydrates as fuel. This

---

will leave you feeling tired, grumpy, and sloth-like toward the end of the day. Those with large amounts of HSL burn fat all day and look thin and slim. Those without it grow fat throughout their adult years.

Thus, if you're consuming Diet Coke you are shutting down your body's ability to burn fat by inhibiting HSL! This inhibition of HSL due to sweets (like aspartame and diet coke as a whole) will occur regardless of what kind of diet you are on. It may also interfere with the use of fat burning supplements currently on the market.

Diet Coke is a joke. Stay away from it and other sugar sources if you're serious about losing fat and keeping it off. Remember, obesity is killing 800 people per day in America!

Principle 4 – Drink 16 ounces of water before every meal

Drink water and you will burn more fat by activating thermogenesis. A proven, simple, yet effective technique that is often overlooked is water consumption. Boschmann and associates from Humboldt University, utilizing a technique known as whole-room indirect calorimetry, have shown that drinking water does, in fact, activate your body's natural ability to burn fat. To be more precise, it was found that drinking 500 ml (16 ounces) of water in one sitting increased metabolic rate by a whopping 30%![199]

The thermogenic effect of water should be used by every man, woman and child. To do this, 500 ml or about 16 ounces of water should be consumed 5 minutes before every meal. This will ensure that you do not overeat and that excess

---

[199] Boschmann, M. et al. "Water-induced thermogenesis." *Journal of Clinical Endocrinology and Metabolism.* 2003 Dec; 88(12):6015-9.

calories are consumed via heat production rather than being stored as fat.

Principle 5 – Whey Isolate and Micellar Casein Protein

It has been shown that different foods can stimulate thermogenesis more than others, most noticeably protein-rich food. More accurately, up to 30% of protein can be dissipated as heat! This is one of the reasons why high protein meals increase lean body mass. Those who consume protein do not have to exercise to rid their body of the calories, as a good portion of them simply gets dissipated as heat, rather than getting stored as fat. This can be done while watching CNN or football. Hence, it is no surprise that Americans have embraced the high-protein diet with so much enthusiasm, they erroneously believe that eating protein will make them thin without doing anything else. Protein consumption also prevents the increase in weight gain that is common to "yo-yo dieting". And third, consuming protein with meals also helps circumvent the previously mentioned insulin spike. Protein does this by slowing the absorption of food into the bloodstream. This is a most important attribute that should be internalized by those who are overweight, insulin resistant or diabetic.

If you are not supplementing protein, namely whey isolate and micellar casein, then you are not serious about your health. Protein supplementation, next to water, is the most important thing you can do to actively burn fat while at the same time gain numerous health benefits. Just as you regularly purchase bread and butter at the grocery store, you should also purchase a good supplement source of whey isolate and micellar casein (making sure that it does not contain sugar or artificial flavors, see Whey Advanced at www.health-fx.net).

Whey isolate and micellar casein, when used together, are a match made in heaven. Combined, such a protein supplement allows for a quick surge of nutrients into the blood stream, while at the same time allowing for a steady release of amino acids and protein over a longer period of time. This increases satiety and prevents the artificial feeling of being hungry for longer, relative to carbohydrates and fat. Hence, protein supplementation greatly prevents overfeeding. More exciting, protein supplementation activates thermogenesis. This is known as meal-induced thermogenesis.

Utilizing whey isolate and micellar casein will increase fat free mass, reduce fat mass, and improve metabolism. Athletes will be happy to know that such a protein supplement, when combined with carbohydrates, can increase endurance by up to 40% and prevent muscle breakdown by 83% (see www. the-drip.net).[200]

In addition to optimizing fat free mass, protein supplementation also prevents sugar cravings and controls appetite by increasing serotonin levels in the brain. Serotonin is derived from L-tryptophan. Recent studies suggest that whey supplementation naturally enhances brain serotonin levels by increasing L-tryptophan levels by 46-48%! That whey can increase serotonin levels is a result of the whey protein alpha-lactalbumin containing large amounts of the amino acid L-tryptophan. Researchers found that this effect of whey (when supplemented 45g/day for 6 weeks) translated to an increase in cognitive performance among users as could be seen by an increase in learning, attention and memory. Additionally, the increase in L-tryptophan would lead to increased mood, focus and the decline of sugar cravings.

Protein supplementation is not just for those looking to lose fat and control appetite, although who wouldn't want to? It is beneficial for individuals of all ages. While infants need protein for proper growth, adults and elite athletes need

---

[200] *Medicine & Science in Sports & Exercise.* 36, 7:1233-1238, 2004

protein to replace what is lost each and every day from exercise and the body's normal biochemical reactions. Therefore, whether you are a competitive bodybuilder, soccer mom, elite endurance athlete, or health conscious consumer, your body is very much dependent on protein for optimal wellness.

Very few individuals realize the importance of protein supplementation. Supplementing with protein provides an entire array of essential amino acids and biologically active proteins that our bodies cannot make yet are mandatory for life. More specifically, our bodies can only produce 11 of the 20 amino acids that are necessary for living. The body must obtain the other 9 essential amino acids from outside sources such as whey isolate. Essential amino acids are histidine, isoleucine, leucine, lysine, methionine (and/or cysteine), phenylalanine (and/or tyrosine), threonine, tryptophan and valine. All of these are well accounted for in a whey isolate and micellar casein blend.

As we can see, the body has a very unique, life-sustaining relationship with Mother Nature. If the body does not obtain the entire array of essential amino acids, it slowly deteriorates. This deterioration is commonly seen as obesity as well as cancer, fatigue, depression, ADHD (especially in children), high blood pressure, muscle atrophy and Type-II Diabetes, just to name a few! While protein does have important attributes, recommending it does not discount the extreme importance of carbohydrates (low glycemic index carbohydrates).

Sadly, due to 21st century fad diets, processed foods and overuse of prescription drugs, most individuals are not obtaining their body's required amounts of amino acids and proteins (as well as minerals and essential fatty acids). As a result, millions of people are suffering from the aforementioned ailments. Rather than reach for protein supplementation in the form of whey isolate and micellar casein, most reach for FDA approved drugs. This is not without considerable consequence to health and life, as shown in chapter 3.

In closing, one cannot be lazy minded and thin at the same time. Rather than be a slave to your body, take charge by making a conscious effort to follow these 5 principles of activating thermogenesis. Science has unveiled a wealth of knowledge in terms of how to lose fat. It could be said that because of these scientific advances in understanding obesity we have never had it so good. Take advantage of it. Engage your brain daily and use discipline when deciding what you will do to be thin. Remember it is a lifetime process, not a quick fix.

Am I overweight?

Below is a Body Mass Index (BMI) chart. You can use this to quickly determine if you are overweight. Simply identify your height and weight and find the corresponding BMI. A normal weight is a BMI of less than 25; overweight is between 25-30 and obesity is over 30. More than half of Americans have a body mass index of 25 or more!

Body Mass Index

Weight (lb)	5'0"	5'2"	5'4"	5'6"	5'8"	5'10"	6'0"
120	23	22	21	19	18	17	16
130	25	24	22	21	20	19	18
140	27	26	24	23	21	20	19
150	29	27	26	24	23	22	20
160	31	29	27	26	24	23	22
170	33	31	29	27	26	24	23
180	35	33	31	29	27	26	24
190	37	35	33	31	29	27	26
200	39	37	34	32	30	29	27
210	41	38	36	34	32	30	28
220	43	40	38	36	33	32	30

It is important to understand, the BMI is only a general indicator for determining whether or not someone is carrying excess fat. To better determine how much fat and muscle you have there is a simple formula.

Step 1: Step on the scale.

You need a baseline measurement of your weight for figuring out the rest of the formula.

Step 2: Measure your body fat % (BF%).

While there are several ways to accomplish this, one of the easiest and least expensive ways is to use a body fat caliper at your local gym. Otherwise, you can use an online body fat calculator at http://www.health-fx.net/healthcalc.html to get an accurate measure of BF%.

Step 3: Multiply your weight by your measured body fat percentage to find out how much fat you're lugging around. Record your answer for future measurements.

Example: 185 lbs. X 17.5% (or .175) = 32.4 lbs. of fat

Step 4: Subtract the amount of fat (in pounds) from your original bodyweight in Step 1.

Example: 185 lbs. (original weight) - 32.4 lbs. (of fat) = 152.6 lbs. lean weight

This calculation **WILL** tell you how much **LEAN WEIGHT** you're currently carrying. However, this first measurement will **NOT** tell you how much muscle you have since your lean weight is also made up of bones, organs, hair, etc.

What it **DOES** give you is your baseline measurement to compare with future measurements since any gains you make in **LEAN** bodyweight should only come from **MUSCLE.**

Step 5: Perform Steps 1-4 again approximately 3-6 weeks later. Then compare your results with your previous reading.

Example: Let's say your first measurements were...

Weight - 187 lbs.

Body fat % Reading - 17.5%

187 x 17.5% = about 32.7 lbs. of fat

187 - 32.7 = 154.3 lbs. lean bodyweight

Now, for your second measurements you get...

Weight - 190 lbs.

Body fat % Reading - 16%

190 x 16% = about 30.4 lbs. of fat

190 - 30.4 = 159.6 lbs. of lean bodyweight

If you now compare your second readings with your first, you can see that.

You've **GAINED** 5.3 lbs. of muscle (from 154.3 lbs. lean in first reading to 159.6 in the second); and you've **LOST** 2.3 lbs. of fat (from 32.7 lbs. of fat in first reading to 30.4 lbs. in the second).

Closing

This book is not an attack on western medicine. In fact, the latest technology in emergency medicine has been an asset to the longevity of human life. Endeavors made by emergency room doctors are admirable and heroic to say the very least. Their dedication to saving human lives often goes unrecognized, as emergency room doctors perform miracles daily.

This is an attack on the ignorance and greed of the American people; including doctors, patients, and pharmaceutical companies. The reliance on drugs, surgery, and high-tech equipment to treat our unwillingness to take responsibility for our own health is killing us, and according to the aforementioned statistics, most of us will overdose on FDA approved drugs before we will ever need the expertise of an emergency room doctor.

Our health has become a stomping ground for greedy drug companies. The lackadaisical attitude toward health among most Americans has driven drug companies and medical doctors to label everyday occurrences as disease, while profiting immensely. Like an item for sale, most have sold their health for miracle drugs and false promises. As a result, in the 21st century, true health is not a right, it is a privilege.

The privilege of health is only bestowed upon those who not only seek the truth, but also, using their free will, act on it. If not acted upon, accept the fact that you will forever become an asset to the pharmaceutical industry who, admittedly and with open arms, will profit from your lack of health.

Quoted from O.S. Marden, true health has been called "the great multiplier of ability, the buttress of initiative, of courage, of self-confidence, the backbone of enthusiasm, without which nothing worth while was ever accomplished." True health is so valuable that if you have it, you wouldn't trade it for all the money in the world. Innately we know this, and because of its value, most are giving their lives and money away for false promises made by pharmaceutical companies.

Obtaining good health relies solely on YOU. Your belief is the most powerful medicine. Lack of belief in your health will always manifest itself into poor health… Believe in your health and you will begin taking part in habits that will attract wellness, both mentally and physically. After all, it is habits that create and eradicate disease, not FDA approved drugs.

Resources

Health Myths Exposed Website
www.healthmyths.net

SafeTaste Certification (TM)
www.safetastecertified.com

The SafeTaste Certification (TM) seal was designed to educate consumers on tastes that kill and tastes that heal.

Nutritional supplements for fat loss, prevention of heart disease, longevity and sports performance
www.health-fx.net

Sports nutrition for endurance athletes
www.the-drip.net

Acetyl-L-carnitine (ALCAR) and alpha-lipoic acid (ALA)
A properly formulated stack of these nutrients can be found under the trade name LifeFX at www.health-fx.net

Natural health education
Global Institute For Alternative Medicine: www.gifam.org

GIFAM offers holistic continuing education programs for nurses through the convenience of distance learning.

Global College of Natural Medicine: www.gcnm.com

GCNM offers home study programs in Nutrition, Herbal Medicine and Holistic Health for busy adults throughout the globe.

Scientific Research
www.pubmed.com

Alternative cancer treatment information
www.cancure.org

International Advocates for Health Freedom (IAHF)
www.iahf.org

Vaccine information
www.thinktwice.com

Stevia Extract for Quitting Sugar Forever
www.stevitastevia.com

Cooking with Stevia
www.cookingwithstevia.com

Vaccine Exemption Forms for ALL States
http://blogs.cloud-busters.com/messiahmews

Index

apoptosis 85
Aredia (pamidronate disodium) 46
Arimidex (anastrozole) 46
Aromasin (exemestane) 46
arrhythmia 12, 117
articular cartilage 72
ASCOT-LLA 124, 131
aspirin 61, 62, 127, 133, 137, 149, 160, 177, 179
atherosclerosis 91, 101, 102, 103, 104, 106, 110, 114, 116, 140, 143, 144

B

B12 95, 114, 117, 132, 144
Baycol 15, 127
beta-carotene 93
Bextra 61
bioactive peptides 95
blood clots 46, 47, 116, 141
BMI 10, 45, 171, 193
Body Mass Index 45, 171, 193
brain damage 30
breast cancer 27, 46, 85, 137
Brown Adipose Tissue 173
bupropion. *See* Wellbutrin, Zyban
Bush 51

C

cachexia 81
cancer 28, 33, 45, 61, 74, 81, 82, 83, 84, 85, 86, 87, 88, 89, 91, 95, 97, 118, 119, 124, 128, 130, 134, 135, 136, 137, 144, 150, 171, 180, 191, 200
CARE 125, 130, 137
CDC. *See* Center for Disease Control
Celebrex 36, 59, 60, 61, 62
Center for Disease Control xv, 8, 41, 95
CHD. *See* coronary heart disease
checkbook science 58, 64, 65, 67
chemotherapy 45, 81, 82, 84, 85, 86, 87, 89
cholesterol 12, 24, 25, 26, 50, 71, 98, 101, 102, 103, 104, 105, 106, 107, 108, 109, 110, 111, 112, 113, 114, 116, 117, 118, 119, 120, 121, 122, 123, 124, 125, 126, 127, 128, 130, 132, 134, 135, 136, 137, 138, 139, 166
Claritin 34, 35
Climera 26, 27
Clinoril 61

SSRI. *See* Selective Serotonin
     Reuptake Inhibitor
statin 24, 25, 26, 106, 107,
     108, 109, 124, 125,
     126, 127, 128, 129,
     130, 131, 132, 133,
     134, 135, 137, 138,
     139
statins 24, 25, 106, 107,
     108, 109, 120, 123,
     124, 125, 126, 128,
     131, 135, 138
statin drug trials 124, 126,
     130
stevia 185, 186
stroke 25, 30, 45, 46, 47,
     84, 102, 116, 117,
     130, 131, 138, 142,
     145, 150, 154, 155,
     159, 163, 164, 165,
     171, 184, 185
sulindac. *See* Clinoril

T

Tamoxifen, (Nolvadex) 46
Taxol (paclitaxel) 46
Taxotere (docetaxel) 46
thermogenesis 173, 174,
     175, 176, 177, 178,
     179, 181, 186, 188,
     189, 190, 192
The Advisory Committee
     on Immunization
     Practices 7

The American Association
     of Poison Control
     Centers 51
The Drug Enforcement
     Administration 9
The Pure Food and Drug
     Act 1
Tolectin 61
Tolerability 56
tolmetin. *See* tolmetin
Toradol 61
transient global amnesia.
     See loss of memory
tremors 9, 31

U

UFT. *See* Uracil-tegafur
Uracil-tegafur 88

V

valdecoxib 61
vascular endothelial growth
     factors (VEGF) 137
violent behavior 4, 5, 30
Vioxx 61, 62, 84
Vitamin A 93
vitamin C 91, 95, 108, 115,
     132, 141, 142
vitamin D 95
Voltaren 61

W

Weight gain 44
Wellbutrin 10, 11, 12, 45,
     157

About the Author

Shane is a graduate of Fort Lewis College. Continuing his academic career he obtained a Master's degree in organic chemistry from Northern Arizona University. During his graduate career he studied the design and synthesis of amino acid and peptide derivatives for use in the asymmetric synthesis of diaminosuberic acid (DSA). DSA is a novel tool which medicinal chemists use in the growing field of peptidomimetics. In contrast to conventional medicine, peptidomimetics offers increased effectiveness via selectivity and safety in the field of medicine.

Abandoning a career in corporate drug making, he is now an independent researcher and consultant to both athletes and the nutritional supplement industry. He is responsible for designing numerous safe and effective nutritional supplements for longevity, fat loss and sports performance. He is also the developer of the SafeTaste Certification (TM) seal, designed to educate consumers on tastes that kill and tastes that heal. He is a member of THINCS, The International Network of Cholesterol Skeptics. Shane is a proud husband and father.

Feedback for this book can be sent to healthmyths@safemail.net

Printed in the United States
25376LVS00001B/133-135

9 781420 800272